Developing Your Career
in Nursing

Developing Your Career in Nursing

Edited by
Desmond F.S. Cormack
RGN, RMN, DIP ED, DIP NURS, MPHIL, PHD

Honorary Reader in Health and Nursing
Queen Margaret College, Edinburgh

CHAPMAN AND HALL

LONDON • NEW YORK • TOKYO • MELBOURNE • MADRAS

UK   Chapman and Hall, 11 New Fetter Lane, London EC4P 4EE

USA   Chapman and Hall, 29 West 35th Street, New York NY10001

JAPAN   Chapman and Hall Japan, Thomson Publishing Japan, Hirakawacho Nemoto
            Building, 7F, 1-7-11 Hirakawa-cho, Chiyoda-ku, Tokyo 102

AUSTRALIA   Chapman and Hall Australia, Thomas Nelson Australia, 480 La Trobe Street,
            PO Box 4725, Melbourne 3000

INDIA   Chapman and Hall India, R. Sheshadri, 32 Second Main Road, CIT East,
            Madras 600 035

First edition 1990

© 1990   Chapman and Hall

Typeset in 10 on 12pt Palatino by
Best-set Typesetter Limited, Hong Kong
Printed in Great Britain by
T.J. Press (Padstow) Ltd, Padstow, Cornwall

ISBN 0 412 32130 0

British Library Cataloguing in Publication Data

Developing your career in nursing.
  1. Nurses. Professional education
  I. Cormack, Desmond F. S.
  610.730711

  ISBN 0–412–32130–0

Library of Congress Cataloging in Publication Data

Developing your career in nursing / edited by Desmond F.S. Cormack.
        p.   cm.
    Includes bibliographical references.
    ISBN 0–412–32130–0
    1. Nursing—Great Britain—Vocational guidance.   2. Nursing—
Vocational guidance.   3. Career development—Great Britain.
4. Career development.   I. Cormack, Desmond.
    [DNLM: 1. Career Choice.   2. Clinical Competence.   3. Education,
Nursing, Continuing.   4. Nursing.   WY 16 D489]
RT82.D47   1990
610.73'06'9—dc20
DNLM/DLC
for Library of Congress   90–1478
                                                                   CIP

Contents

Contributors

Philip Barker RNMH, PHD Clinical Nurse Consultant, Royal Dundee Liff Hospital, Dundee

David Benton BSC, MPHIL, RGN, RMN District Research Nurse, North East Essex Health Authority, Colchester

Robert Cooper BA, RGN, RFN, RCT, RNT Deputy Director of Nurse Education, Highland College of Nursing and Midwifery, Inverness

Desmond Cormack RGN, RMN, DIP ED, DIP NURS, MPHIL, PHD Honorary Reader in Health and Nursing, Queen Margaret College, Edinburgh

Julia Coxon BA, RGN, RM, NDN, HV Tutor's Certificate Lecturer, Department of Health and Nursing, Queen Margaret College, Edinburgh

John Hodgson MA, LLM (CANTAB), SOLICITOR (HONS) Senior Lecturer in Law, Nottingham Polytechnic, Nottingham

Patricia Peattie BSC (SOC SCI), RSCN, RGN, CMB PT1, CERT ED., RNT Principal, Lothian College of Nursing and Midwifery, Edinburgh

John Tingle BA LAW (HONS), MED, Barrister, Senior Lecturer in Law, Nottingham Polytechnic, Nottingham

Preface

Each registered nurse, midwife and health visitor is accountable
for his or her practice, and, in the exercise of professional
accountability shall:. . . take every reasonable opportunity to
maintain and improve professional knowledge and
competence. (United Kingdom Central Council for Nursing,
Midwifery and Health Visiting, 1984, p. 2.)

This statement responds to the self-imposed requirement of the nursing profession which expects that members will satisfy the above criterion. It indicates that each registered nurse is personally responsible for maintaining and improving professional knowledge and competence. Nurses are well suited to respond to this part of the UKCC Code of Conduct. As well as having a long tradition in meeting self-imposed professional expectations, nursing has developed a sophisticated infrastructure with which to continuously develop and update skills and knowledge. Although there is a personal responsibility to undertake this activity, a high quality and quantity of support systems exist. In part, this process is helped by investing some personal time and energy in systematically planning and developing a career. In addition to contributing to meeting the requirements of 'professionalism' the purpose of planning a career is to optimize its quality, and the extent to which it contributes to personal/professional satisfaction and development.

Developing Your Career In Nursing may include, but is by no means restricted to, planning for progression through a series of promoted posts. Development is equally necessary for those who, for any of a number of reasons, decide not to progress up the promotional ladder, but who wish to continue to work in existing positions as clinicians, managers, teachers or researchers; or who reach some other stage beyond which promotion is not sought. This book is intended to provide a structure within which to make decisions about how a career can develop, throughout the course of that career.

Professionals become expert by virtue of knowledge, skill, experience and attitudinal change. Career development enables fulfilment of potential in relation to expertise at all levels. It facilitates the provision of direction and leadership to peers and less experienced colleagues. For example, the person who has a special expertise in working with dying children, or in caring for people suffering from dementia, fills a leadership role which enables others to learn from that expertise. Means by which this leadership function can be optimized includes systematic career development.

Although the major function of pre-registration training programmes is to produce able and safe clinicians, these programmes also focus on the development of a career beyond registration. I hope this book will contribute to the consideration of this area, and assist teaching staff to make the subject an integral part of students' professional awareness.

In addition to those general chapters which discuss the nature of, and need for, career planning/development, others are included which examine specific aspects of career development such as writing, research, reading, job applications and preparing a curriculum vitae. These specific chapters are not intended to teach how to become 'expert' in those areas; rather, they are designed as a starting point from which to develop these particular components of successful career development. The range of topics is not exhaustive; they are presented as examples of the kinds of issues which might be considered. For example, if a gap in relation to understanding of research is recognized, the chapter on that subject will assist in making good that deficiency. The quality of the contribution which can be made by nurses is strongly influenced by the way in which career development is planned. Personal contribution to health care can be optimized by planning individual career development in the context of health care generally, thus making use of the contribution which other groups can make to the development of nursing, and to individuals within it. This assertion is equally relevant to clinicians, administrators, researchers and teachers.

The content is relevant to those who are presently undergoing initial training. It is widely recognized that exposure to such a concept is an integral part of such an education. *Developing Your Career In Nursing* presents a structure and content for dealing with this part of the syllabus. It is also intended that the text will be of value to qualified staff who are considering means of structuring their career development; either in the context of a post-registration course or as part of on-going independent study.

The term 'nurse' is used throughout the text in a general way which is intended to include all those who have a nursing background/training, and who are currently working in an area which requires the use of nursing knowledge and skill.

Some parts of the text have a more immediate application than do others although, in the long term, all are of importance. Because of the varying time-frame which it addresses, some parts are written in the more immediate (present) tense, others in the future tense. Some parts of the text have a relevance for the 'here and now', others will be of more value as a career develops in later years.

In the short term virtually all nurses become clinicians, in the longer term some will become teachers, managers and researchers. As the general principles underlying career development are the same for all groups. I intend the book to be of use whichever career path is taken.

Developing Your Career In Nursing as a whole, and its individual chapters, are neither comprehensive nor exclusive. The whole, and its parts, are designed to introduce a concept which will lead to a personal initiative in terms of maximizing personal contribution to, and rewards from, a career in nursing.

Throughout this text, nurses will be referred to as 'she'. This convention will be used as a matter of convenience, and fully recognizes the equally important contribution of men in nursing.

Desmond F.S. Cormack

REFERENCE

United Kingdom Central Council for Nursing, Midwifery and Health Visiting (1984) *Code of Professional Conduct for the Nurse, Midwife and Health Visitor* (2nd edn) United Kingdom Central Council for Nursing, Midwifery and Health Visiting, London.

Part One

Chapter 1

Nursing career development

DESMOND CORMACK

On becoming a student, the first major step is taken in developing a nursing career. Indeed, it can be said that career development started well before training began, when nursing was selected and the appropriate entry qualifications obtained. This pre-entry phase is the 'springboard' upon which all other parts depend. Training provides a necessary and important foundation for developing the ability to personally contribute to, and obtain satisfaction from, a nursing career. Cox (1984) described registration as the beginning of professional development. As a result of becoming a student there exists the requirement and opportunity to give attention to the way in which a career develops throughout its life-span. Sale (1987), who saw the strong links between personal, professional, and career development suggested that: 'Personal development means different things to different people but in general terms it is taking responsibility for your own actions...' (p. 5).

In addition to providing an essential base from which to plan a career, pre-registration education provides the focus for planning short-, medium- and long-term career development goals following qualification. For example, training may include some exposure to research, career opportunities, job applications and the functions of professional organizations. Although, of necessity, the emphasis is on clinically-oriented matters which serve to make proficient practitioners, much is also done which provides an excellent basis for continuous career development.

WHAT IS CAREER DEVELOPMENT?

Career development is the means by which individual contributions to nursing and health care generally are maximized. It is also the means by which the highest level of personal and professional satisfaction is reached. It encompasses a variety of education inputs and career pathways (Owen, 1985). Career development optimizes what is obtained from, and given to, the profession, and contributes to the quality of all aspects of nursing practice, teaching, management and research.

Nurse education, which is prescribed and closely monitored by professional bodies, prepares effective, safe and proficient clinicians, that being its primary purpose. Inevitably, such an education cannot effectively prepare for the remaining ten, twenty or forty years of a professional life. At best, it can be seen as giving an initial preparation for working at a reasonably effective, safe and proficient level (Sweet, 1986). Subsequently, other factors begin to play a central role in, and make demands on, a nursing career. Those additional factors include experience and continuing career development.

Experience

Experience comes as a natural consequence of 'doing the job' for which nurse training provided a basis, the quality of that experience being influenced by the way in which it is used. There are two positions which can illustrate the point. First, one experience might provide fewer opportunities for building on and developing initial education, causing the individual to function without fully extending and continuing that education. Such an experience would be less likely to encourage acknowledgement of those areas of educational experience which were deficient, thus placing the nurse at risk in terms of 'stagnating' and being overtaken by events in a short space of time. The second (more usual) position is one in which the experience is innovative and challenging, causing the individual to recognize how much more needs to be learned in terms of skills and knowledge. Such a recognition is likely to be followed by continuous involvement in the means of making good these deficits.

By merely working in a particular area and gaining 'experience', a partial contribution to career development is made in terms of quantity. However, if that experience is not complemented by quality, the point of diminishing returns is soon reached when additional experience (of the same kind) contributes less and less to professional development.

Figure 1.1 presents a model ('divergent outcome model') which serves two purposes: first, it traces the 'value' of experience over an imaginary time-frame; second, it illustrates the relationship between experience and career development. The model suggests that the early part of a new experience (A) consists of a necessary period of adjustment when little 'new' material is assimilated. This, and all other parts of the experience, are enhanced by concurrent career development activity. The adjustment period is followed by accelerated learning phase (B). A 'plateau' phase (C) follows, during which time much of value is learned over an extended period. Finally, the 'divergent outcome period' (D) has two alternative outcomes depending on whether or not the experience has been accompanied by concurrent career development activity. The first alternative (————) results in a decrease in the value of experience if that experience

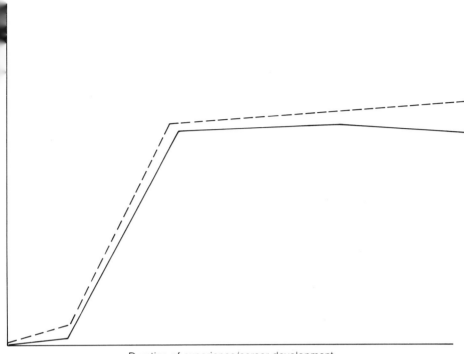

Duration of experience/career development

A	B	C	D

⟨ . . . . . . ⟩(. . . . .)(. . . . .)(. . . . . ⟩

Figure 1.1 Experience/career development relationship (divergent outcome model). A, adjustment period; B, accelerated learning; C, learning plateau; D, divergent outcome period. ⎯⎯⎯value of experience only; ------ value of experience + career development.

is not accompanied by concurrent career development activity. The second alternative (-----) results in an increase in the value of experience if that experience *is* accompanied by concurrent career development activity.

Continuing career development

Professional training is both the basis of, and an integral part of, a nursing career, as is the quality and quantity of clinical experience. There is a further factor which contributes to a career and to professional development generally; that factor is continuing career development. By this is meant the way in which training and experience are added to by

systematically building onto professional skills, knowledge and understanding. This is a process by which the ability to contribute to personal
and professional areas of functioning are extended and expanded. In some
areas the benefits are shared by an employee and employer, for example a
successful job interview. In others, patients reap the benefits, for example,
because of nurses' understanding of the latest research. It may be colleagues who gain, by an ability to inform them via publishing for instance.
It may be the profession which has the advantage of individual contributions to issues and debates of professional importance. Finally, it may be all
of these individuals and groups who benefit.

However, none of these outcomes of career development are separate,
they are all closely linked aspects of the way in which contributions to, and
satisfaction derived from, a career are maximized.

IS CAREER DEVELOPMENT NECESSARY?

The answer is a very definite 'yes', it is an integral and necessary part of
all professions, including nursing. Such are the great number of factors
relating to career development about which choices can be made, the
possibility of success can be increased by making the best choices. Although 'chance', 'luck' and 'being in the right place at the right time'
influence a career, it can be more positively influenced by conscious
decision-making and planning (Manthorpe, 1985, 1986). This approach
does not consist of a rigid plan for the future which cannot be altered
to take account of changing needs, resources and circumstances. On the
contrary, career development is a dynamic process with sufficient flexibility to take account of unforeseen events, and of changing needs and
circumstances. There are, however, some aspects of development about
which there is less choice. For example, there is no choice in relation to
reading the professional literature; to do so is part of the notion of
professionalism. The degree of choice, and subsequent flexibility, lies in
deciding what to read.

In considering the question 'Is career development necessary?' the term
'career', which can be used in two ways, requires clarification. First, it can
be used to describe a long-term commitment to working in nursing. This
might take a number of forms such as spending a working life-time in the
level/grade entered following registration; or refer to progressing up a
promotional 'ladder'. The second use of the term includes promotion in
either clinical work, teaching, administration or research (or a mixture). In
this text, the term 'career' encompasses both definitions, it refers to the
professional and personal development of anyone with a long-term commitment to nursing, and who may or may not wish to achieve promotion
from the position entered following registration, or from their present
position.

WHEN SHOULD CAREER DEVELOPMENT BEGIN?

The obvious answer is that planning started some time ago, probably well before the decision was taken to become a student nurse. A choice was made to enter nursing, to obtain the necessary educational qualifications, and to enter a chosen course. Prior to training, a decision may have been made concerning the clinical specialty, or specialties, in which initial and subsequent experiences would be obtained. During training, decisions may have been made regarding the types of post-registration courses to be taken. Consideration may also have been given as to whether a future career will focus on clinical work, teaching, administration or research, or on more than one of these. A pattern of professional reading will have started, decisions about which journals to buy or borrow will have been made. Thought will have been given as to trade union and/or professional organization membership.

The aim of this book is to provide a structure within which a life-long commitment to career development can develop. The nature of professionalism involves taking on these responsibilities. The answer to the question 'When should career development begin?' is 'At the beginning of the career, if not earlier'. Just as plans were made for beginning a career, plans for ending it, often by retirement, must also be made. All points between the beginning and end require attention.

HOW IS A CAREER DEVELOPED?

Career development starts with the recognition that it requires and responds to systematic short-, medium- and long-term planning. Although these plans are dynamic, they provide a structure and direction to that development. Some aspects have been implemented on entering nursing and/or a particular specialty. Initial training provides much of the basis for the future. However, plans also require to be made for subsequent development and for continuing the momentum provided by initial training.

The clinical focus of training includes, of necessity, a partial introduction to non-clinical aspects of career development. The starting point, therefore, is to take stock of which career development skills and knowledge (in addition to initial training) already exist. Such a self-evaluation will enable the identification of areas of strength, relative weakness, and those in which more knowledge and/or skill are required.

Priorities are then identified, enabling short-term and long-term goals to be set. For example, if limited time is currently devoted to reading the professional literature, this can be made good in the very short term. Conversely, if additional involvement in contributing to the professional literature is required, that goal might be set for the medium term. Some subjects may be identified as being much less relevant to a particular career. For example, if there is no immediate intention of obtaining a new job, then job search and interview skills require little attention. However, since all other aspects of career development contribute to success in job search and interview, provision for that eventuality is naturally being made.

A greater or lesser amount of time may be available for career development during working hours. For some, there is encouragement and opportunity to read and write professional material at work, for example. For others, less encouragement and opportunity exists. This implies that more or less 'personal' time has to be spent contributing to professional development, something which may be difficult in some circumstances. However, opportunities can be taken to make use of even limited time in which to develop in the areas discussed in this book. The rewards from investment of time and energy are substantial in that a career *develops*; maximizing contributions to, and satisfactions from, that career. The resources and opportunities available for career development are varied and considerable. During the past two decades, the professional literature, educational opportunities, funds for career development, and the quantity and quality of highly skilled resource persons have increased dramatically. Better local, national and international lines of communications have enabled increased use to be made of the knowledge and skills which lie outwith a particular locality. There now exist numerous formal commitments by various professional organizations, statutory bodies and employers to help individuals develop their career. Indeed, some organizations are now employing a 'career development co-ordinator'.

Recently, a colleague asked how she might prepare for a job interview. She was an experienced person who, in addition to her job, had successfully undertaken looking after a home and bringing up a family of three. Like some other nurses (both male and female) with a variety of personal and domestic commitments, she had spent many years in her profession without taking much account of a number of important wider issues which might reasonably be regarded as key features of career development. A previous (unsuccessful) job interview was discussed, an experience which had left her frustrated and disillusioned by her recognition of a poor interview performance. She said that she had been unhappy about the quality of her replies to a number of interview questions, and wished to discuss how to improve her performance. Examples of the questions were:

'How do you keep up to date with your specialist area?'
'Have you any views on report X?' (a recently published report of considerable importance to her specialty).
'What plans do you have for developing your career during the next few years?'
'Which key issues are currently being debated in your specialist area?'

'How have you organized your continuing education since qualifying?'
'Which research articles/reports have you read recently?'
'Do you read any professional journals on a regular basis?'
'Which professional libraries do you use?'
'Who are the people you would regard as leaders in your profession?'
'What do you understand by the term "professionalism"?'

In the previous job interview, she admitted that she had found it difficult to give constructive or meaningful replies to these questions. She felt that she had never fully considered these issues as being of relevance to her, a position which may have been partly influenced by the fact that her training, which was undertaken a number of years earlier, did not prompt her to fully address these issues on a continuous basis.

Subsequent to our meeting she decided to withdraw the application for the job for which she was soon to be interviewed, a decision prompted by the recognition of a number of knowledge/skills deficits. At a later meeting, a number of short-term career development goals were identified which would help to make good these deficits before submitting a job application at a later date. In short, she belatedly recognized the importance of continuous career planning and development.

It is not suggested that all job interviews contain questions of the type in this example, although they are appropriate and relevant in interviews for any level of nursing position, and are being more frequently addressed. Indeed these are issues which are part of a full career development, whether or not a job interview is anticipated. In short, they are a constant part of professionalism, the ability to address them constructively and positively being an integral part of a professional career.

CONCLUSION

A number of items for inclusion in subsequent chapters have been selected, a selection which, to some extent, reflects personal preferences and interests. This selection points to the fact that there is no 'recipe' which can be applied to all individuals and circumstances; undoubtedly there are a number of other issues which contribute to a successful career development.

Some parts of the book are more relevant to the short term or medium term, others are more relevant to the long term. For example, reading professional literature is a necessary part of development which begins during training, and continues throughout. Also, writing for the professional literature becomes more important as experience is gained. However, the base from which writing skills are developed is professional education and experience. Thus, writing-for-publication skills start to develop as soon as one became a student nurse, although they are most often used later in a career.

Career development issues should be considered as early as possible (Bates, 1986), and exist within the context of the role of the qualified nurse having clinical, managerial, teaching or research elements, and, according to Weeks and Vestal (1983), should assist movement between these career paths.

REFERENCES

Bates, A. (1986) A square peg in a round hole. *Senior Nurse*, **5**(4), 30–1.

Cox, C. (1984) Structured professional development. *Nursing Mirror*, **158**(19), 35–7.

Manthorpe, D. (1985) Your career in nursing: The options. *The Professional Nurse*, **1**(3), 65–7.

Manthorpe, D. (1986) From student nurse to D.N.S. *The Professional Nurse*, **1**(5) 134–5.

Owen, R. (1985) Professional development — Is it your business? *Nursing Practice*, **1**, 40–2.

Sale, D. (1987) *Professional Development for Nurses*, Health Services Manpower Review, Mercia Publications. Keele.

Sweet, B.R. (1986) From the first day of the rest of your career. Continuing education of the midwife. *Midwives Chronicle*, **99**(1185), vii–ix.

Weeks, L. and Vestal, K. (1983) PACE: A unique career development programme. *The Journal Of Nursing Administration*, **13**(12), 29–32.

Chapter 2

Transition from student to professional

PATRICIA PEATTIE

BECOMING A STAFF NURSE

All the ambition which brought about an application for nurse training has finally culminated in successful achievement of the goal — to be a nurse. Nothing can quite compare to those first days of wearing a staff nurse uniform, really doing the job of a professional practitioner in your own right — so why do you, as a new staff nurse, so often feel unprepared, anxious and ill-at-ease? Henderson (1969) noted that:

> The unique function of the nurse is to assist the individual, sick or well, in the performance of those activities contributing to health or its recovery (or to a peaceful death) that he would perform unaided if he had the necessary strength, will or knowledge, and to do this in such a way as to help him gain independence as rapidly as possible. (p. 4)

Virginia Henderson's well-known definition of a nurse may well be the conceptual framework within which you as a learner nurse identified the role of the nurse. The ambition, or the desire to become a nurse, may have arisen in early childhood. It may have been nurtured by supporting friends and relatives and life expectancies, or may have been sustained in the face of adverse comment and events.

Most candidates for nurse training express a wish to care for people. It may well be, especially for the young applicant, that the precise nature of the activities involved are hard to identify, the stresses and strains of the role ill understood, and the professional responsibilities and scope on qualifying unknown. On the other hand, some applicants are older, rich in life experience, may have tried other occupations, gained academic qualifications in other disciplines and turned to nursing as a means of personal fulfilment. Certainly it seems unlikely that anyone enters nursing with a view to having an easy life, with good pay and regular hours. Social changes have improved pay and working hours, but still there is the shift system and weekend working essential to the provision of a 24-hour service to be considered.

Training programmes vary considerably across the country, but all seek, within their national requirements, to prepare a practitioner who is safe to practise as a registered nurse.

This aim might be expressed in more detail as enabling the nurse to:

- care for the individual patient or client according to his individual needs
- manage and co-ordinate the nursing and health care of groups of patients/clients
- apply theoretical knowledge to practical situations
- devise nursing care plans based on observation, knowledge and critical judgement according to observed and perceived needs
- become a full member of the health care team with a vital contribution to make to any therapeutic action
- develop her own unique approach to nursing care and initiate action where necessary
- be competent in nursing skills
- be able to pass these skills to others
- use her intellectual, practical and social skills to improve and maintain standards of care, and continue to develop and practise these throughout her professional life.

It is important not to over-emphasize the level of competence expected of the newly qualified nurse. You are *not* the expert — yet. It may well be that some of the disillusionment and indeed depression and disappointment experienced by many nurses in the early post-qualifying months, arises from their own, and others', unrealistic expectations of their role on qualification.

Stress and role strain

The experience of nurse training and education should enable the nurse on registration to begin to learn fully the business of nursing. However, because the notions of 'becoming a nurse' and 'being a nurse' are closely related to the training process and ultimate qualification, it may well be that the practitioner feels she has arrived when she registers, rather than just begun her professional journey. The months of hard work leading to the examinations, the wait for the results and the exhilaration on receipt of the pass letter, fade in the face of new job anxieties.

In addition, the staff nurse role, which is usually the first post-qualifying post, is not well defined. It is seen as being an inferior form of charge nurse/sister when the designated senior nurse is not on duty, or reverting to the senior student role when patient care needs demand this. To the newly-qualified nurse, the difference between the role of staff nurse and that of charge nurse/sister is not clear. She therefore tends to use that of the charge nurse/sister which is, in fact, inappropriate, being a different role with different responsibilities and authority.

Change is always a threat to internal security. As the years of training progress, and appropriate skills, knowledge and attitudes are acquired, each movement from one ward to another becomes easier, the settling down process takes less time, and the increasing confidence derived from this measurable progress further reduces anxiety. However, moves to very specialized and different areas (for example, theatre or the community) may still create stress because the degree of change is greater and there is commonly an assumption that little of the learning previously acquired can be usefully transferred. The major change of status and function on becoming a staff nurse is inevitably accompanied by anxiety.

Whilst some anxiety can be a stimulus, with senses alert and attention increased, undue anxiety can reduce attention and narrow the perceptions. Severe anxiety can cause stress symptoms which reduces the capacity to concentrate on more than fine detail to the exclusion of other, important concerns. Such a state cannot be in the interests of patients or the practitioner, so individuals must take steps to reduce undue anxiety by careful planned preparation for new roles.

In many ways, the additional knowledge and professional awareness makes the later transitions more fraught with stress and anxiety, whether these be into new areas of practice or from the one level of responsibility to another within the same area of specialism (Chapter 4).

Additionally, the career change may be accompanied by other stressors, such as a house move into a strange town, a new health board as employer, personal life changes and demands. Role conflicts not previously experienced may arise for the first time, coinciding with the initiation into full professional status as a qualified nurse, accountable for the actions of herself and others.

Many new staff nurses tend to feel adequately prepared for their clinical role in the organization and delivery of direct patient care, though this confidence is not always shared by tutors and sisters who know them. However, far less confidence is expressed about certain types of relationships, such as communicating with doctors, and dealing with dying patients and their relatives. The managerial aspects of the job, therefore, seem to pose the major problems and these views were reflected in a research study by Lathlean (1987 a,b).

Some of the difficulties for newly qualified staff lie in uncertainty of the role, the responsibilities, the level of authority and the degree of accountability the individual has. You may be experiencing this ambiguity yourself as you begin your first job as a staff nurse.

At the time of registration, a copy of the United Kingdom Central Council for Nursing, Midwifery and Health Visiting (UKCC) (1984) Code of Professional Conduct for the Nurse, Midwife and Health Visitor is sent to each nurse. This outlines the standard of professional practice against which individual behaviour should be measured to determine professional conduct. It underlines the essential nature of professional practice as respecting the client above all, and behaving at all times in a manner which instils public trust and confidence. It also confirms the individual professional practitioner's accountability for her own practice.

Professional accountability

In the past, nurses have not been particularly encouraged to be accountable for their practice. They have shouldered immense responsibility, often exercised considerable authority, but avoided accounting for their actions. Too easily have nurses yielded inappropriately to the pressure from others to conform or to cope, or accepted the readiness of other professions to direct their practice.

Several factors are involved in individual accountability (Figure 2.1). First, the nature of the charge (or task or activity) needs to be clearly identified and understood. Second, the individual must have the abilities to carry out the charge. Third, the individual must be given and accept the responsibility for the charge, and finally, have the authority to do so.

How does the newly qualified nurse consider these issues? Training may have clarified your early views of the business of nursing and it may have prepared you to deliver high standards of direct patient care. However, for many new staff nurses, there appears to be a gulf between their concept of the role for which training was apparently designed to prepare them, and the reality which they find on appointment. Many of the skills acquired in training appear to be rarely utilized, and many of the skills which the new role demands appear to have been ignored in even the 'management' block or module.

THE FUNCTION OF THE NURSE

Perhaps this is the first time, without the pressure of examinations directing reading and thoughts, that you can seriously address the question 'What is nursing?' and perhaps equally importantly 'What is not nursing?'. From these deliberations it should be possible to assess the nature of the charge and clarify whether or not a particular activity is part of the nursing function.

Nursing is a caring role, and nurses can and should interpret this widely but with discrimination. Nurses do not have the monopoly in caring, but exercise it in a particular sphere. The caring activities involve individual patient care, the overview of nursing care given by a team, and the administrative duties which facilitate the meeting of care needs.

Much has been written, and many debates held, about the extended role

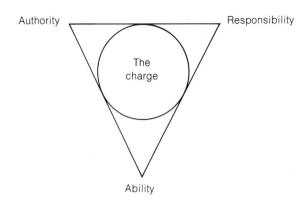

Figure 2.1 Individual accountability.

of the nurse. It may well be that tasks previously carried out by others who now find themselves overstretched could properly become the business of suitably trained nurses. Such an acceptance of a new 'charge' might well enhance the care of the patient who has a particular need, and may improve the smooth running of the area, reducing irritation and frustration arising from interruptions in nursing activity. However, it is not a nursing activity to relieve the pressure on other professional practitioners at the risk of reducing the capacity of the nursing team to fulfil all the nursing functions effectively. It is often easy for nurses to be subject to emotional blackmail, as all activities impinge to some extent on patient well-being, but it is important for each nurse to analyse her ideas of the nature of nursing and the real reasons why a particular charge should, or should not, be accepted. Some tasks, by virtue of having previously been the responsibility of doctors, or of having a 'high-tech' profile, appear to give nurses status if handed on to them, and may be eagerly absorbed into regular nursing activities. Equally, other activities may appear to be non-nursing duties, easily carried out by clerical or domestic staff. In the past, some quite crucial nursing functions have gone outwith nursing control on this basis.

Both these approaches are inappropriate. Some nursing activities are hard to define and defend, and it is likely to be these which go to the wall when other more overt activities become a nursing function. By not retaining some of the more apparently mundane activities within the nursing role, the opportunity for discrete observation and informal uncontrived communication which can form the basis for so much decision-making, is lost.

For example, is it really appropriate for nurses to accept responsibility, even with appropriate additional skills training, for technical tasks such as venepuncture, inserting intravenous cannulae or organizing the priorities of admissions? Such tasks may relieve doctors of time-consuming work, when they are already overburdened and from which they could justifiably be released. But if this additional burden passes to nurses who are already having difficulty in meeting patient need for the comfort of a quiet chat or listening ear, it is not an appropriate use of the available resources.

On the other hand, to have limited involvement in admitting non-emergency patients, or in the serving of meals reduces opportunities for patient contact which may impair assessment for care and evaluation of progress. Also, there is a real risk that this delegation of activity may become an abdication of responsibility with a consequent reduction of authority and control.

Naturally, people like to be liked, and want to get on well with other people working in the same environment. Indeed, it is in the spirit of the UKCC Code of Professional Conduct (1984) (Clause 5), that specific efforts should be made to work co-operatively and collaboratively with others in the multi-professional team. However, this has to be balanced by the equally important injunction, expressed in Clause 10, to consider factors which may place patients in jeopardy, or militate against safe standards of practice.

Skills and decision-making

The next issue for the nurse to review is the question of the abilities required to fulfil the charge. On selection for nurse training, consideration is given to all the attributes a person has already, as well as the assessed potential for development. These are built on and enhanced during the planned training programme to enable the individual to practise as a nurse. No one enters nursing as a blank slate, nor are they, at the point of registration (or ever) 'finished' nurses. Somehow, many nurses seem to feel that they must know everything, never be in doubt, never be seen to ask for help or advice, for fear of being deemed unable to cope and judged incompetent.

You must be capable of an accurate assessment of your own intellectual, practical and affective competencies. You must also be able to identify your own limitations, and take steps to improve and develop your skills. Simultaneously, in any particular work setting, you must be capable of assessing the requirements for the particular charge in question so that appropriate delegation within the nursing team is exercised and appropriate help and advice sought when necessary.

For the newly-qualified nurse, this aspect of assessing the skills of others, especially student nurses, and matching these abilities to the care needs and supervisory skills available can be a difficult task. It may be helpful to rethink the purposes of assessment which are to:

- reinforce good practice and increase motivation
- correct error and diagnose problems
- provide feedback between teacher–supervisor–student
- counselling
- certification (final judgements resulting in recommendations for an award or qualification).

It will not be possible for senior nurses to prevent unsuitable students entering the profession unless each assessment is honestly and objectively completed, and all these purposes borne in mind.

To make these decisions, when in doubt, nurses should turn to other nurses for advice about the business of nursing. As students, there seems to be little hesitation in asking for help and guidance from nursing colleagues, both student and trained staff. Perhaps this is in recognition of the student role in relation to the nursing team, and the right of senior staff to direct and control nursing activity. The same attitudes should prevail when you become qualified. Now the point of reference will be the next most senior nurse on duty at the time, that is, using the line management, or tapping the skills and knowledge of more experienced nursing colleagues working in other areas.

Accepting responsibility for the charge implies a recognition that abilities match the need. Both individually for a specific task, and collectively for a whole ward workload, this requires careful consideration.

For many new staff nurses, the matters of direct patient care for individuals may pose few problems. The managerial concerns are, however, new. Empty beds there may be, a patient may undoubtedly require admission, but can the workforce meet the additional demand without jeopardizing safe standards of care for others, or their own health? Is the new admission really better off just by physically being in the ward, or is everyone merely lulled into a sense of false security until something goes wrong and it is clear that patient safety has been put at risk? Physical overcrowding, inadequate resources; these are the proper concerns of the nurse. The nurse must be able to use cogent argument to protect patient and staff safety based on objective assessment of the situation. Too often nurses have argued from an emotive standpoint: it may well be that anger, frustration and other emotions influence the decision to take a stand. However, the successful outcome of such debate is more likely if the nursing viewpoint is put forward factually, calmly and firmly, recognizing the weight and value of other viewpoints and the implications for the nursing professional practice if these other views eventually determine the decisions reached.

The desire to have problems resolved speedily to reduce patient distress may persuade an inexperienced nurse to accede to requests to carry out unauthorized functions, for example giving medication not prescribed in writing, not getting things checked, or other shortcuts. These things, however well intentioned, may none the less endanger patient safety and thereby risk the professional practice of the nurse.

Sphere of staff nurse authority

Accepting responsibility for a charge having acknowledged that the abilities are available to fulfil it can only be sound if you also have the authority to do so. Authority for particular spheres of activity may be written into the job description and may be clearly described or merely implied. Health Board policy statements may also specify spheres of authority, and each nurse should be clearly aware of her employing authority's policy statements. Authority for particular actions may also be enshrined in statute and the registered nurse needs to be familiar with those aspects of legislation of relevance to her work (Chapter 6).

Spheres of accountability

Having given careful consideration to all these issues, a professional practitioner can be expected to be accountable. You are accountable first and foremost to your patients for the delivery of professional standards of nursing care. You are also accountable to your senior managers for the maintenance of standards of care in your area of practice and for your own professional practice. You are accountable to the other members of the team for your part in the collective effort and for the effectiveness of the nursing functions. You are accountable to your professional colleagues for your own professional development and the furtherance of nursing knowledge and competence. Finally, you are accountable to yourself for self-discipline, maintaining and delivering high standards of practice without the close and constant supervision experienced whilst a student.

The professional practitioner also has a responsibility to ensure that practice is safe in terms of the current state of knowledge. This is changing rapidly, partly due to the speed of medical and technical advancement, and to the development of nursing research. Nursing research is increasingly providing a sound, scientific basis for making nursing practice decisions. Other writings describe the developments of nursing theory which can assist in planning care appropriately for individual patients. It is the business of every nurse to endeavour to understand and apply the new knowledge on the basis of a critical analysis of its worth. This development of skill will demand further education and opportunities for debate should be actively pursued by each practitioner (Chapter 8).

Nursing practice encompasses a number of very different roles, all of which have to be performed in ever-changing circumstances. Over the next few years, nurse training will change considerably, and the education process will promote in nurses the skills and qualities to meet the challenges of the next century. However, these practitioners will present a challenge to current practitioners, who may feel threatened unless each one accepts the responsibility for her own professional development.

The registered nurse as clinical practitioner

All nurses are practitioners, but a mistake is often made by nurses themselves and others, in interpreting that concept as the 'hands-on' task-centred function, for example, giving medicines, assisting with hygiene needs. This clearly cannot be a definition of nursing: many friends and relatives, and patients themselves, maintain high standards of practice in these kinds of activities (and indeed in some others which might be the province of only a few nurses, for example, renal dialysis).

The true difference between the professional nurse and unqualified caregivers must be in the ability to assess need as it changes and adjust plans to meet their needs, choosing from a wide range of nursing strategies the most appropriate. Equally, the registered nurse must be capable of developing finely tuned assessment skills to identify individual differences so that individually tailored holistic care can be implemented. This should encourage the scientific evaluation of nursing practice, thus providing evidence for continuing with, or rejecting, a particular approach. It is these decision-making and observational abilities, with their implications for a knowledge and skills base, an analytical approach and flexible attitude, that justify the nurse as a professional practitioner.

However, one aspect of practice that has often received little opportunity for skill development during training is related to stressful situations with patients and their relatives. Such occasions are not for a crowd; bereaved relatives, or patients coming to terms with a poor prognosis, are often dealt with by the senior nurse in a private manner. This may be quite appropriate, but it does mean that a newly qualified staff nurse faces such a situation for the first time, unsupported. When anxious, it is all too easy to feel that 'something must be said' and yet the words don't come and silence appears a mark of professional incompetence. Perhaps more nurses need to learn how to use silence as a comfort, to recognize the value of touch, of 'being there', and of listening. It is also necessary to strive to provide means of enabling learners to feel more competent in these distressing situations by involving them in some aspects of the comforting role to reduce their feelings of inadequacy on qualifying.

However, because these skills and abilities are not merely theoretical, the clinical setting is the place in which novice practitioners acquire them. Thus the registered nurse is a role model for learners, whether they be supernumerary or part of a paid workforce. The need to create a good learning environment is the responsibility of the permanent nursing staff in any ward. Taking care to clarify expectations, to give clear instructions, to delegate appropriately, to explain and support practice, to teach new skills, and listen and respond to questions, will all reduce learner anxiety and thus increase patient safety. The way in which work is allocated so that these conditions can be met is shown to be the single most important factor in creating a good learning environment.

A truly supportive approach, readily adopted in any setting, is to pair junior and senior nurses and allocate work on the basis of groups of patients. Certainly, a more holistic approach is more common now than in the past, but it is still fairly rare to observe this taken to the point of assessing the skill mix to meet the needs of patients. The possibility of giving responsibility for caring for the same patients over a period of time should also be considered. Not only can the constant changing of areas of responsibility cause anxiety to the patient and reduce communication, but the loss of opportunity to get to know patients affects the comparative, qualitative nature of observations carried out by the nurse.

The nurse as teacher

Teaching may be seen to be the prime responsibility of specialist practitioners at a more senior level. However, just by being there, you *are* teaching: how you look, how you perform your duties, the attention you pay to details, which issues are perceived to be important and whether the reasons are understood and accepted will all enhance or detract from your influence as a teacher. The learning will take place: each practitioner has the personal responsibility to ensure that it is not bad practice that will be observed and emulated.

A consequence of the involvement of learners in the practice area is the need for them to be assessed, given encouragement to sustain good practice, and motivation to improve where skills are lacking. One major difference between the expert and the novice is that an observer of the practitioner at work can clearly see the confident, smooth, effective practice of the expert whether or not a full understanding of the job exists. Obviously, therefore, the unskilled learner will be slow, will be unsure, and will lack confidence. This must be taken into account when planning the work, so that anxieties are not unduly caused, and patient safety put at risk.

Nurses need to be more willing to give praise where it is due and also to assess in an objective manner so that poor practice can be identified and suitable corrective strategies devised. Ultimately, so that unsuitable practitioners are not permitted to continue in training, the professional nurse must be prepared to provide objective evidence, written down and signed on the assessment forms.

For the new staff nurse, so recently the subject of this assessment process, it can be difficult to criticize the practice of others, especially senior students only months junior in experience. The problem is compounded by the unclear expectations particularly in relation to the professional attributes rather than practical skills. It is true that, even when some attempt has been made by the educational establishment to provide guidance in this area, both by a suitable form and some opportunities for discussion, these judgements have a major subjective element in them. It is a responsibility of the registered nurse to endeavour to protect patients from unsafe practitioners and this can only be achieved if individual nurses do not avoid taking unpleasant decisions. If praise is given when due, and clear supporting evidence provided for adverse judgements, some difficulties can be avoided and confident appraisal achieved.

The nurse as manager

Standards of practice need to be identified as part of the management function of the nurse. Goals in terms of appropriate patient care cannot be achieved unless consideration is given to the identification of relevant resources, both of personnel and equipment. Increasingly, managers at ward level will be accountable for the budget, and no successful bargaining will be achieved if the ward stocks are inappropriately maintained and other resources squandered.

Within the management function comes the consideration of priorities. It is never going to be possible to achieve the ideal for all, even if it were known what that might be. There is always a mismatch between skills and resources available and the demands on the service. Hard decisions have to be made about what is possible. If what is possible is also an unacceptable outcome for patient care then that must clearly be demonstrated to senior management, whose responsibility it then becomes (UKCC Code of Professional Conduct (1984) Clause 11).

The registered nurse must also be able to communicate with the nursing team effectively. This involves the consideration of the nursing activities, and the rationale underlying the decisions upon which plans are based, so that a truly co-operative effort is achieved and she in turn receives from colleagues the information and support necessary for her to act as the nurse member of the multi-disciplinary team in an effective manner.

As an equal member of the multi-disciplinary team, you must be prepared to take an active part in decision-making. The nursing care of a patient is her responsibility, but she must also ensure that its results — the information gleaned in conversation, the objective data collected and recorded, and any anxieties or difficulties that the nurses are aware of, are brought to the team's attention and fully discussed. The patient must be enabled and encouraged to put forward his/her viewpoint and if this is not possible, the nurse must recognize her responsibility to be his/her advocate.

ETHICAL DILEMMAS

All members of the team have a professional responsibility towards the patient, which implies that all will seek the patient's good, and act in what they believe to be the patient's best interests. None the less, in many situations, it will be unclear what the best course of action should be, and only if all the different professional perspectives and that of the patient or relatives are equally considered, is it likely that a suitable way forward can be found.

Many of these issues will indeed be hard to solve. There are real ethical dilemmas facing practitioners every day. Whilst it is clearly a responsibility of the medical practitioner to prescribe medical care, it is a team matter, including the patient and relatives, if the question of 'treatment with what or at all' is an issue.

To contribute fully to this complex debate, and in order that patients, relatives and colleagues may place trust and confidence in the professionalism with which decisions will be reached, each individual must explore for herself the basis upon which moral decisions are reached in her own life. Once you have this self-knowledge, and recognize the need for re-examination as life experiences alter perspectives, you can identify your own views and biases, and recognize possible areas of conflict in your future work.

It is not essential necessarily to change your views, although some beliefs and values may be incompatible with continuing practice as a nurse. It is, however, essential that every patient receives care to meet his physical, emotional and spiritual needs without fear or favour, accepted for what he is and able to be fully confident that his care is in his best interests.

True professionalism is hard work, is not achieved lightly but is a necessary goal for every nurse to gain the respect of professional colleagues and the public, so that the nursing care afforded to the patient is of the highest standard within a dynamic service.

Many nurses, in the past, felt that the end of training was the end of studying, the end of books. Nurses, traditionally, did not read, or consider that they needed to meet colleagues outside official working hours, for debate or consultation. As a result of increasing complexity of care needs and the greater awareness of the need for continuing education, attitudes are slowly changing. Each registered nurse must take personal responsibility for keeping up-to-date, having a flexible approach to practice and be willing to give personal time to professional development.

The first step on the road is to learn the role of the staff nurse — it is an exciting, challenging time, and one which can have the greatest influence on patient outcome. The staff nurse is closely concerned with direct patient care, has the ear of senior colleagues in the multidisciplinary team and the opportunity to contribute to the development of the profession by the quality of her own work and the supervision and guidance offered to learners and unqualified staff.

The successful career depends on forward planning, each step carefully considered to keep as many options open as possible. Regular reviews of your developing strengths and skills will enable suitable choices to be made. The remainder of this book may give you some more ideas of possible directions which will lead to a satisfying career. The passport has been earned; the journey has still to be planned, prepared for — and enjoyed!

REFERENCES

Henderson, V. (1969) *Basic Principles of Nursing Care*, International Congress of Nurses, Geneva.

Lathlean, J. (1987a) Are you prepared to be a Staff Nurse? *Nursing Times*, **83**(36), 25–7.

Lathlean, J. (1987b) Prepared transition. *Nursing Times* **83**(37), 42–7.

United Kingdom Central Council for Nursing, Midwifery and Health Visiting (1984) *Code of Professional Conduct for the Nurse, Midwife and Health Visitor*, (2nd edn) United Kingdom Central Council for Nursing, Midwifery and Health Visiting, London.

FURTHER READING

Burnard, P. and Chapman, C.M. (1988) *Professional and Ethical Issues in Nursing. The Code of Professional Conduct*, Wiley and Sons, H.M. & M., Chichester.

Downie, R.S. and Calman, K.C. (1987) *Healthy Respect. Ethics in Health Care*, Faber and Faber, London.

National Consumer Council (1983) *Patient's Rights*, Her Majesty's Stationery Office, London.

Royal College of Nursing (1989) *Exercising Accountability*, Royal College of Nursing, London.

Runciman, P.J. (1983) *Ward Sister at Work*, Churchill Livingstone, Edinburgh.

Thompson, I.E., Melia, K.M. and Boyd, K.M. (1983) *Nursing Ethics*, Churchill Livingstone, Edinburgh.

Chapter 3

Individual professional assertiveness

DESMOND CORMACK

The focus of this chapter is on the concept of individual assertiveness, with some reference being made to aggression in its positive form. The latter term is, unfortunately, largely used in its negative form in the nursing literature in that it is usually used interchangeably with the term 'hostility'. In an attempt to clarify the meaning of these terms, *Collins English Dictionary* (1985) defines '*Assert*...to insist upon (rights, claims etc.)...to put oneself forward in an insistent manner', 'dogmatic or aggressive'. '*Aggressive* ...assertive; vigorous' '*Vigorous*...endowed with bodily or mental strength or vitality; robust...'.

The use of these terms, and the way in which they are defined, invite confusion in both writers and readers. In this text the terms assert/assertion/assertiveness relate to insisting upon rights and to putting oneself forward in an insistent manner, the term 'aggressive' will relate to being assertive or vigorous. The positive use of the term 'aggressive' and its close relationship with assertiveness is demonstrated by a statement recently made by a nursing director during an interview on radio. In reply to the question 'What type of nurses are you trying to recruit?', she replied: 'We need, bright, able and aggressive nurses. These are the people who can ensure the best quality of patient care.' The positive use of 'aggressive' is frequently made when describing successful salesmen, athletes, business men/women and a range of professionals who function in an assertive and vigorous manner.

Assertiveness therefore, is the ability to insist upon personal rights (whilst recognizing professional responsibility and accountability) and to put oneself forward in an insistent manner, and having the mental strength, vitality and professional background to do so. It is a combined function of the individual, and of a professional confidence which results from appropriate education and experience.

Although changing, the tradition of nursing is not firmly based on individual assertiveness. Rather, nurses and nursing have been perceived as being relatively submissive. However, as the science of nursing grows and generates a professional education which produces individuals who base decisions, actions and arguments on a greater degree of scientific/objective principles, assertiveness will cease to be an issue in nursing. It will become the norm which nurses, nursing, consumers, other health care disciplines, and society will expect, even insist on. The recent changes which illustrate increasing assertiveness include the development of the nursing process, the movement toward a nursing model of care which requires greater autonomy and accountability, the introduction of primary nursing, increased research activity, the movement into higher education, the ability of nurses to write for publication, and to speak/debate in public. In relation to midwives, Cronk (1988) stated: 'A midwife is required and trained to exercise her clinical judgement. . . . She is further directed to take note of research in her field and to be responsible for her own professional development.' That statement emphasizes the need for individual clinical assertiveness based on a full awareness of current research, and on an adequate level of personal professional development. A similar assertion was made by Dainow (1986) who commented that assertiveness springs from the philosophy that every individual was responsible for what he or she did.

FACTORS INFLUENCING/INFLUENCED BY INDIVIDUAL ASSERTIVENESS

Figure 3.1 demonstrates the inter-related nature of the factors which influence and are influenced by assertiveness in the individual nurse. The process is a cyclical one which has no fixed starting or end point. However, in order to illustrate how the process might influence (and be influenced by) student entrants, that starting point will be used (I). Although the model focuses on entrants to initial nurse training, it also has relevance to those who are undertaking post-registration education, in the course of which a realignment of personal assertiveness is achieved.

I Student entry

On entry to nurse training, a student has a number of preconceptions regarding the relationship between nursing and assertiveness. For example, one belief might be that nursing is a subservient profession which reacts to the direction and leadership of other professions, or that individual registered nurses react to the expectation and directives of others in the nursing hierarchy. Such a person may have little understanding of individual professional rights, responsibilities and autonomy. It may be that their recruitment to nursing, via a selection process which discriminates in favour of compliant/submissive entrants, perpetuates the myth of non-assertiveness being a desirable quality. Thus, it is possible for nursing to attract recruits who are seeking a profession in which they

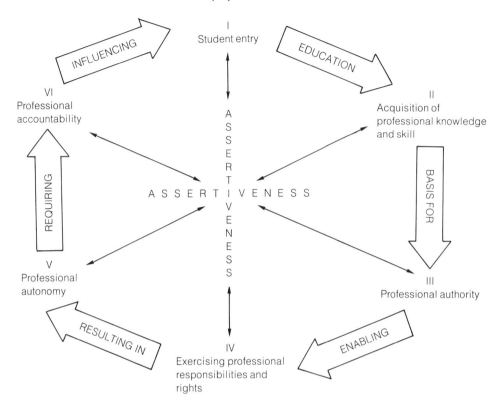

Figure 3.1   Factors influencing/influenced by individual assertiveness.

will be led rather than lead, in which decisions will be imposed rather than personally made, and in which there is a relatively low expectation in terms of individual assertiveness and responsibility. If entrants are being recruited into a profession which is low in the submissive/assertiveness continuum, and by selection panels which have a similar orientation, this will be reflected in the personality of the successful entrants.

A quite different position will exist when the profession, and individuals within it, are perceived as being assertive, autonomous and valuing the ability to lead and make decisions based on the notion of professionalism, and accompanied by an appropriate level of professional knowledge and skill. Such a profession will attract assertive recruits who are willing to play an active (assertive) role in professional decision making and practice. The same principles apply to nursing practice, management, education or research. Selection of students for entry into nursing, and for places on post-registration courses, will clearly be influenced by the relatively assertive orientation of selection panels who will positively discriminate in favour of applicants with a similar orientation.

The educational background and ability of entrants will also influence the extent to which they will adopt a submissive/assertive professional role. As will be seen in the discussion of part II, much depends on the ability of the individual to acquire a level of professional knowledge and skill which, in addition to enabling the provision of an appropriate quality of care, will become a foundation for responding to professional responsibilities and rights, and for developing professional authority and autonomy.

II   Acquisition of professional knowledge and skill

Nurse education, which rightly provides a balance of knowledge, attitudinal change and skill, includes a substantial breadth and depth of material which makes considerable intellectual demands on students. Traditionally, nurse training focused on what nurses should do, rather than on why, and was based on a reactive rather than proactive approach to care. The relatively recent focus on why nursing is performed in a particular way has caused much of traditional nursing to be challenged, evaluated and, on occasions, altered. The proactive approach has caused nurses to anticipate nursing needs, rather than respond to those which are identified by others.

Although new entrants to the profession are increasingly encouraged and expected to be assertive in their expectations regarding their education (including the extent to which they learn from clinical experience) there is evidence to suggest that some of their trained colleagues in clinical areas are resistive to that notion. Chudley (1988) described the instance of a student nurse who started training following completion of a university degree. She reported that in the university she was used to an environment which nurtured questioning, and a thinking and changing approach. Following commencement of nurse training, the same nurse reported that she had moved to an environment where these qualities were positively discouraged. A similar point was made by King (1988). Although the assertive (including questioning) individual may be perceived as threatening to senior colleagues who are passive, insecure or who have some other reason for maintaining the *status quo*, nursing is increasing in professional maturity and confidence to the extent that acceptance of assertive individuals is becoming the norm rather than the exception.

Assertive approaches to nursing, embodied in the changing focus of nurse education, are encouraged by the type of education which causes nurses to question, make informed decisions, and recognize professional responsibilities and rights which lead to professional authority and assertiveness. Such an education recognizes that students cannot be taught how to deal with all circumstances on all occasions. In addition to providing the basis for professional functioning, contemporary nurse education equips the nurse to continue with a personal/professional development which will extend the ability to make informed and independent decisions. Finally, the education and subsequent development will enable the nurse to explain and justify decisions and subsequent actions, it will have assertiveness as a natural and appropriate consequence and will provide the basis for the development of professional authority.

III   Professional authority

Authority has been defined as the power to control, judge or inhibit the actions of others (Hanks, 1985). This definition applies to that which is exercised in an organization such as nursing, with 'senior' clinicians or managers, controlling, judging or inhibiting the actions of others (subordinate) staff. The type of authority is also referred to as 'structural authority'. Another form of authority (professional authority) is that which has been referred to by the Committee on Senior Nursing Staff Structure (1966) as 'sapiential authority' which they defined as: '. . . the right, vested in a person, to be heard by reason of expertness or knowledge — just as one person, relative to another may be an ''authority'' on a particular subject' (p. 117).

Professional (sapiential) authority, therefore, is that with which the professional nurse is invested by virtue of the acquisition of a specialist body of nursing knowledge and skill. The result of acquiring this knowledge and skill, accompanied by a prescribed amount of experience, is that the individual becomes the authority on nursing. This form of authority applies equally to the nurse clinician, manager, teacher and researcher. It has equal relevance to the individual nurse and to the nursing profession generally. As professional experience increases, accompanied by related career development, a corresponding increase in the individual's level of authority is achieved. Thus, the professionally educated nurse is the 'authority' in all matters relating to nursing which are within her sphere of influence, and which are based on previous education and experience. This authority carries the responsibility and right of the nurse to be assertive in conveying it to other nurses, to colleagues from other health professions, and to making use of it in relation to nursing practice, teaching, management and research.

IV   Exercising professional responsibilities and rights

The professional responsibilities of nurses are described in the codes of professional conduct which have been prepared by a number of national registering bodies. Such a code has been published by the United Kingdom Central Council For Nursing, Midwifery and Health Visiting (1984). The apparent overt focus of such codes of conduct is on the clinical aspect of the nurse's role, with frequent references to patient/client's care, safe standards of practice, and conditions or safety of patients/clients. However, such codes, by implication, also relate to nurse teachers who are preparing nurses to meet the requirements of such codes, to nurse managers who provide the resources necessary to meet these requirements, and to nurse researchers who interact directly with patients and who contribute to the knowledge base from which clinicians, teachers and managers comply with such codes.

Professional assertiveness is implicit in many, if not all, parts of the code of conduct which apply to all registered nurses, midwives and health visitors in the United Kingdom (United Kingdom Central Council For Nursing, Midwifery and Health Visiting, 1984). The code of conduct contains similar elements to those constructed by, and relating to, nurses in other countries. Individual assertiveness is required to enable compliance with such a code of conduct in order to: 'Ensure that no action or omission on his/her part or within his/her sphere of influence is detrimental to the condition or safety of patients/clients' (p. 2), and 'Have regard to the environment of care and its physical, psychological and social effects on patients/clients, and also to the adequacy of resources, and make known to appropriate persons or authorities any circumstances which could place patients/clients in jeopardy or which militate against safe standards of practice' (p. 3).

These examples, two of fourteen items contained in the UKCC Code of Professional Conduct, require nurses to have a professional education which will provide the knowledge, confidence and ability to ensure that an appropriate quality of care is provided, and to take steps to make known circumstances which militate against safe standards of practice.

Professional rights are implicit in all parts of the UKCC Code of Professional Conduct, and are explicit in others. The code gives the individual the right to function in the manner described in each of its parts, most of which relate to the interests of clients/patients, others applying to the individual nurse (UKCC). For example, the nurse has the right to: 'Take every reasonable opportunity to maintain and improve professional knowledge and competence' (p. 2), and be able to: 'Acknowledge any limitations of competence and refuse in such cases to accept delegated functions without first having received instruction in regard to these functions and having been assessed as competent' (p. 2), and to: 'Work in a collaborative and co-operative manner with other health care professionals...' (p. 2), and to: 'Make known to an appropriate person or authority any conscientious objection which may be relevant to professional practice' (p. 2).

It is not being suggested that such codes of professional conduct contain items which address either responsibilities or rights, but rather that they confer both upon the nursing profession and its individual members. Acceptance of these professional responsibilities and rights becomes the basis of, and results in, professional autonomy, and accountability.

V Professional autonomy

Individual professional autonomy is closely related to individual professional assertiveness. In personal terms, it is clear that some individuals are more assertive (and therefore autonomous) than others. This aspect of personality will cause some nurses to seek and secure their personal rights and to exercise their professional responsibilities, it will cause others to play a relatively passive role. This individual variation in assertiveness levels is normal within any group and applies to all professions including nursing. One aspect of this issue is on the extent to which individual assertiveness contributes to the profession. The greater the degree of individual professional assertiveness, the greater the degree of assertiveness (and collaborative autonomy) in the profession as a whole. By autonomy one means a large degree of self-government, self-determination, and the freedom to make individual and collective nursing decisions. It is realized that no individual or profession can be entirely autonomous; both being required to take account of the views and needs of other professional colleagues, other professions, society and patients.

Nursing is a developing profession which, until recently, was often seen as being subservient to, and largely controlled by, other parts of the health care system generally, medicine in particular. Elms and Moorehead (1977) wrote: 'Nurses have been alternatively envisioned as dedicated old maids cloistered from reality in residence halls, sex symbols endowed with exotic curative powers, and servants administering to the needs of the doctor.' A decade later the notion of nursing being perceived as subservient to medicine was discussed by Smith (1987) and Jones (1987). Indeed, the issue has, and continues to be, the focus of many contributions to the nursing literature. One possible reason for lack of professional autonomy and its equivalent professional assertiveness in nursing is that the profession, and individuals within it, have been prevented from exercising their due rights and responsibilities. When looking for the 'cause' of this problem it is usual to lay the blame at the door of the medical and other professions. The following anecdotes, all derived from personal experience, illustrate the folly of assuming that the nursing profession holds no personal responsibility for the extent to which its professional autonomy has been, and is being, threatened.

1. *At an international meeting attended by over 3000 nurses, a speaker addressed the issue of individual and collective professional autonomy in nursing. She proposed that individual nurses (and the profession generally) were being denied autonomy because nurses, the majority of whom are female, were being dominated by doctors of medicine, most of whom are male. The proposition met with virtually total agreement and applause.*

I am personally sceptical of the view that autonomy in nursing depends on the extent to which others (including the medical profession) wish to *give* autonomy to nursing; that view is a myth. The reality is that autonomy is acquired, rather than given by others.

2. *At a recent series of lectures regarding the long-term care for the hospitalized elderly, two speakers presented independent papers which addressed relationships between nursing and medicine from the perspective of professional autonomy. The first speaker described how he and his nursing colleagues were inhibited from implementing progressive forms of nursing care because of a lack of interest on the part of the consultant geriatrician who rarely visited the ward. The speaker implied that the presence and interest of a medical colleague was necessary for the implementation of high quality nursing care. The second speaker described a similar ward which was regularly visited by an enthusiastic and involved consultant geriatrician. The speaker then clearly indicated that the close attention which the consultant gave to patient care generally, and to the provision of nursing care, prevented the nursing team from providing the type and quality of care which they wished to deliver.*

Although each speaker may have been presenting a reasonable point of view, and highlighting the need for appropriate levels of nursing/medical collaboration, it might also be concluded that a lack of assertiveness/ autonomy would have existed whatever the level of interest and support made available by the consultant medical staff. Additionally, a professionally assertive nursing team should be expected to ensure the presence of an 'absentee' consultant, whilst not allowing such an absence to interfere with the quality of nursing care. Similarly, a nursing team should be able to determine the type and quality of nursing care whilst working with an enthusiastic and involved medical colleague.

3. *During a clinical team meeting which the writer attended with a student nurse as part of a teaching experience, a consultant psychiatrist made a number of conclusions regarding the medical treatment of a patient who was the subject of the case conference. The ward sister, who had been fully involved in the discussion, posed the question: 'What about nursing care?', the question being directed to the psychiatrist. He replied 'What do you suggest?' Following a period of silence, the psychiatrist offered a number of suggestions for nursing care, these being accepted by all the nurses present at the meeting including the sister.*

I am not suggesting that all nurses take a subservient role in relation to care generally and to nursing in particular, nor that they expect other professionals to take the initiative. However, I do suggest that nursing exhibits a sufficient amount of self-imposed subservience (lack of assertiveness and autonomy) to make the issue worthy of debate. The examples given above, in my view, illustrate that lack of autonomy in nursing is related to how nurses perceive their role and is not necessarily externally imposed. The following anecdote illustrates the increasing level of assertiveness (and autonomy) which is developing in nursing.

   4. *Recently a nurse submitted a research proposal for consideration by a local research committee. Prior to its consideration by the committee, the nurse learned that the research committee had no nurse member with a research background. Believing that the proposal could only be appropriately evaluated by a committee which included a nurse with a research background, and being of the opinion that the work of the committee would be enhanced by such a nurse member, the researcher who submitted the proposal successfully negotiated the appointment of a permanent nurse member, who had a research background, to the committee.*

These anecdotes are intended to illustrate the variation which exists within nursing in relation to professional assertiveness and autonomy. They are also intended to illustrate that, contrary to popular belief, the extent to which nurses are autonomous or otherwise is not entirely dependent on external factors. In my view there exists no 'conspiracy' to deny individual nurses, or the profession generally, the right to exercise professional assertiveness, authority, responsibility, autonomy or accountability. Neither medical colleagues, other health care professions, patients or society have the ability or the wish to do so. These aspects of professionalism are not in the gift of any external agency. Rather, they are within the grasp of individual nurses, and the profession generally, if there is an ability and desire to exercise them. There is much to suggest that nurses and nursing have the desire, and are developing the ability, to do so.

Nurses' autonomy is limited to the extent to which they are accountable to their peers, other professionals, professional bodies, to society generally and, of course, to individual patients. Oliver (1988) observed that: 'One of the hallmarks of a profession is the implicit acceptance by its members of the principle of accountability.' Thus, nurses are obliged to account for, explain and defend their actions or inactions, and provide satisfactory explanations and/or reasons for these. The professional nurse is relatively autonomous, there being no such thing as absolute professional autonomy. Where actions do occur without prior consultation and/or permission seeking, they are always influenced by the known views of others, the norms of the profession, and by professional codes of conduct. Thus, the individual takes an action which is felt to be appropriate at that time. To that extent, the individual is acting autonomously. However, all such actions and decisions may subsequently have to be explained and justified as being appropriate and in accordance with what a reasonably competent and informed nurse would have done under similar circumstances. Thus, professional autonomy influences, and is influenced by, professional accountability.

VI Professional accountability

Accountability may be defined as being obliged to account for (explain and defend) one's actions for inactions, and to give satisfactory reasons or explanations for these. The UKCC Code of Professional Conduct makes it clear that 'Each registered nurse, midwife and health visitor is accountable for his or her practice...' (UKCC 1984, 1989).

One of the hallmarks of a profession is the full acceptance of the notion of accountability by all its members. Registered nurses are accountable in law for their actions, to the UKCC, to the consumers of nursing services, and to society generally. Such accountability applies equally to nurse clinicians, managers, teachers and researchers (Chapter 5).

If requested to account for her actions, and found wanting, one of a range of sanctions may be applied, including the possible removal from the Register of the name of the nurse concerned. However, in order to ensure that nurses have the skill, knowledge and resources to comply with the code of professional conduct, the code can be used to draw attention to any of a range of inadequacies which inhibit compliance, and to enable the nurse to refuse to undertake any activity for which she has not been trained.

What makes the professional 'autonomous' is that she has the right to make decisions and take specific courses of action (based on professional education and professional norms) and to be personally responsible for these. The views of colleagues can and should be considered in advance of making decisions and taking actions if there is the opportunity and need to do so. However, professional autonomy places the final responsibility (accountability) for these decisions and actions on the shoulders of the individual, even if these actions have been 'prescribed' by others (Jones, 1988).

CONCLUSION

Assertiveness is being presented as the natural product of the responsibility of nurses to have an appropriate level of knowledge and skill upon which to make nursing decisions, and have the right and ability to implement these. Such a position will recognize the multidisciplinary nature of health care, and the extent to which many decisions overlap and have implications for other professions. Just as the decision of the physician, physiotherapist, social worker and occupational therapist will be made in collaboration with nurses and others in the team, nursing decisions are subjected to the scrutiny of others. Assertiveness, based on appropriate levels of knowledge and skill, and the ability to verbalize these, ensure that decisions relating to nursing practice, management, teaching and research are made by nurses, or with nurses having the primary influence, and are of the best possible quality.

There are situations when the demands of professional assertiveness can contribute to personal stress. For example, if one is, by nature, relatively submissive and dependent, it may be difficult to adopt an assertive professional role. Teaching strategies (Bond, 1988, and the additional articles which were published in the seven subsequent issues of the *Nursing Times*) accompanied by exposure to assertive role models, the presentation of nursing as including professional assertiveness as the norm, and appropriate peer group support can equip the relatively submissive individual to overcome this trait from a professional perspective. Although such teaching strategies may be a useful adjunct to appropriate types of training and continuous career development, they are no substitute for an education and experience which creates professionally assertive individuals. Thus, individual professional assertiveness is synonymous with professionalism.

It may be that this aspect of professionalism (individual assertiveness) has less to do with our inherent worth, than with our ability (or inability) to communicate it to others. Although much has been done in this regard, there remains much to do if we are to fully address this fundamental issue which was described by Schorr (1983) as follows:

> Nurses do magnificent work, yet they are underappreciated, underutilized, underpaid and undervalued. There are many reasons for this condition — but a principal one is that nurses have failed to communicate — to the public, to physicians, to the government, to others, the health care team — an accurate representation of their competence, their professionalism and their potential.

This issue can, and is being addressed, by a continuing increase in individual assertiveness which supports, and is supported by, acquisition of professional knowledge and skill, professional authority, exercising professional responsibilities and rights, professional autonomy, and by professional accountability. This issue can also be addressed by a life-long commitment to nursing career development.

REFERENCES

Bond, M. (1988) Assertiveness training: Understanding assertiveness. *Nursing Times*, **84**(9), 61–4.

Chudley, P. (1988) Glittering prizes? *Nursing Times*, **84**(26), 19.

Committee on senior nursing staff structure (1966) *Report of the Committee on Senior Nursing Staff Structure*, Her Majesty's Stationery Office, London.

Cronk, M. (1988) Midwives must be allowed to exercise clinical judgement (letter). *Nursing Times*, **84**(51), 12.

Dainow, S. (1986) Assertiveness: Believe in yourself. *Nursing Times*, **82**(27), 49–51.

Elms, R.R. and Moorehead, J.M. (1977) Will the 'real' nurse please stand up? *Nursing Forum*, **16**(2), 112–27.

Hanks, P. (ed.) (1985) *Collins English Dictionary*, Collins, London.

Jones, C. (1987) Handmaiden mentality. *Nursing Times*, **83**(40), 59.

Jones, I.H. (1988) The buck stops here. *Nursing Times*, **84**(17), 50–2.

King, W. (1988) A 'trouble-maker' speaks out (letter). *Nursing Times*, **84**(29), 15.

Oliver, G. (1988) Accountability in nursing. *Nursing Standard* (special supplement), **29**(2), 18–9.

Schorr, N. (1983) Communicating for success. *International Nursing Review*, **130**(3), 73–76, Cont. 86.

Smith, L. (1987) Doctors rule, O.K? *Nursing Times*, **83**(30), 49–51.

United Kingdom Central Council for Nursing, Midwifery and Health Visiting (1984) *Code of Professional Conduct for the Nurse, Midwife and Health Visitor* (2nd edn), United Kingdom Central Council for Nursing, Midwifery and Health Visiting, London.

United Kingdom Central Council for Nursing, Midwifery, and Health Visiting (1989) *Exercising Accountability*, United Kingdom Central Council for Nursing, Midwifery and Health Visiting, London.

Chapter 4

Professional stress

PHILIP BARKER

INTRODUCTION

Most of the pressures we experience are associated with psychological and social factors. Apart from demands placed upon us by family, colleagues, friends and wider society, there are stresses associated with our expectations of what we should be doing in various situations. The organization of our lives is also an important source of stress. Many of the demands placed upon us, by ourselves and others, are woven into the 'system' which often directs our lives. Our ability to organize, ourselves and others, can make life less stressful. At times, however, organization makes life more complicated and troublesome, upsetting sleep and eating routines, often with disturbing long-term effects. Nurses are no different from other people in their response to stress. However, some of the circumstances which are stressful for nurses are peculiar to the health-care setting. The nursing environment may be therefore more stressful than other working situations. Stress can be interpreted simply as the situation where demand outstrips the person's ability, real or perceived, to respond to the demand. This is illustrated for a hypothetical nursing context in Figure 4.1. During training, 'demands' and 'ability' may be well matched. In the figure, fluctuating demands are represented by the dotted line and the nurse's 'professional ability' to respond to such demands, by the ascending curve. At various points, the gap between 'demands' and 'ability to respond' widens as when, for example, examinations are imminent, a new clinical problem presents, or the nurse is otherwise 'stressed'. The gap between demand and response acts as an incentive to the nurse to increase her range of skills and knowledge base. On qualification, demands may increase suddenly as the nurse is seen as a fully-fledged professional. New clinical experiences, promotion, increased expectations of others, reorganization and change, are all 'professional events' which contribute to increased demands across time. If the gap between demands and ability to respond widens sufficiently, the nurse may be described as 'over-stressed'. However, the gap can be kept to a minimum by appropriate and continual professional career development.

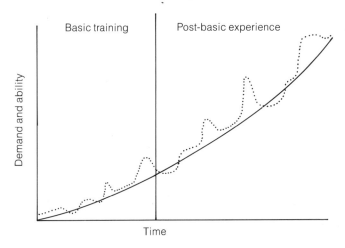

Figure 4.1 The stress gap. Where the level of professional 'demand' and professional 'ability' are closely matched stress is positive. Sudden or sustained increases in demands (such as examinations, threatening clinical situations, new jobs) create stress gaps which are 'distressing'. ———— professional ability; . . . . . . professional demands.

THE NATURE OF STRESS

Not all stress is 'negative'. Selye (1956) distinguished between eustress, or positive stimulation, and distress, which disturbs the individual. Too much (hyperstress) or too little (hypostress) can also have negative consequences. Getting the balance right, especially in a working environment, can be very difficult for nurse managers, researchers and teachers, as well as clinicians. The 'high-tech' environment of the late 20th century has reinforced many of the stressors introduced by the industrial revolution. Noise, artificial lighting and vibration, all produce fatigue in the short-term. Through the disruption of sleep, these can add a further stressful 'knock on' effect in the medium-term. Most people can escape from such stresses only temporarily. Other stresses may be part of our work or life 'style': inadequate or highly processed diets, lack of exercise, inadequate rest, monotonous tasks, enforced inertia and disruptions of our circadian rhythms through shift work or socializing. The effects of such stresses may be delayed, some operating directly on the body (somatic), others through the person, where she 'creates' stress through her interpretation of certain events (psychic). Stress can be defined therefore as the process of transactions in which a person's resources are mobilized and matched against the demands of her environment. The person decides, through a process of appraisal and judgement, how important are such demands, and this is reflected in the bodily resources mobilized to meet such demands. Lazarus and Folkman (1984) noted that where a person's relationship with his environment is seen as 'stressful', it is appraised as taxing or exceeding his resources and therefore endangers his well-being.

Some people are especially receptive to stressors, such as noise, irregularities in circadian rhythms, or demands on the sleep–wakefulness mechanism. Others find it difficult to cope with change in their work situations, or find it difficult to cope with responsibility or decision-making. Consideration needs to be given here to the selection of the care setting in which the individual can best function. The working 'environment', in its broadest sense, includes stressors which have some effect on most people. Shift systems, rest breaks, lighting, heating, work rotas, instructions, equipment, support services, can have a profound effect on individual workers, for good or ill. Where nurses do not have time-out for breaks, work too long under bright or dim lighting, or in a noisy or confined environment, using equipment which is faulty, or inefficient, with inadequate support from other staff, they are likely to become distressed. The source of such stress is in the organization of the clinical setting. Distinguishing between stress as an individual or organizational problem is important for its resolution (Hare, Pratt and Andrews, 1988).

The care setting

Different occupational environments pose different problems. In the clinical situation, for example, this can involve the patient's condition, the nature of the nurse's role, or the organization of care. Where patients are severely debilitated, emotional stress is felt. The nurse who believes she should help everyone towards cure or rehabilitation will find encounters with terminal care or death a distressing experience (Gardner and Hall, 1981). The emotional health of any individual is directly related to the ability to assess and deal with reality. The idea that all patients can be 'cured' or 'rehabilitated' to the same extent is patently unrealistic. What might be a 'good result', for example, where nurses are supporting a child with incurable cancer undergoing chemotherapy, or caring for a severely mentally handicapped child? Setting realistic care goals is fundamental if feelings of impotence or incompetence are to be avoided. Where negative feelings are experienced, it is important that these are openly acknowledged. Nurses have, traditionally, tried to cover up normal emotions, especially those associated with death and dying (Pryser, 1984). Trying to remain emotionally detached, however, conflicts markedly with the advice of psychotherapists who emphasize the need to reveal feelings of frustration, anger and sadness (Parkes, 1972). What is the shame of being human? Some care settings, such as intensive care or transplant units, pose special problems by the nature of the nurse's relationship with the patient. Loneliness can be a very real problem if the nurse is involved with a single, unresponsive patient for several hours (Fromant, 1988). Isolation from the patient can even be experienced where aseptic technique is used on a continuous basis (Pot-Mees, 1987). Perhaps of greatest significance is the technical demands of intensive care where procedures are potentially life-saving (Huckaby and Jagla, 1979) or where the acquisition of new skills are required (Donovan, 1981). Although the sources of stress in such acute clinical care settings are increasingly recognized, little is known of how nurses cope with such pressures (Hague, 1987).

Operating theatre staff stresses are compounded by organizational problems. In particular, changes to operating lists and inefficient use of time affect the nurses' experience of job satisfaction. Effective time management and communication are essential if stress is to be minimized (Astbury, 1986). Senior nurses, often blamed for 'bad organization' or 'inadequate support' to clinical staff, can also be the victims of organizational stress, when 'impossible demands' are made for staffing units, especially at times of high sickness and/or absence levels. Lack of support from their own 'superiors' and exclusion from decision-making can also lead to feelings of resignation and apathy.

Nurses working with disturbed patients, such as the mentally ill (Jones *et al.*, 1987) and people with severe dementia (Athlin and Norberg, 1987), are prone to very high levels of psychological distress. Researchers have emphasized the importance of clear roles, and the support of senior staff, in resolving 'professional depression' (Firth *et al.*, 1987). Where staff are involved with people who might be described as regressed, aggressive, unmotivated, dependent, resistive or incurable, 'psychic stress' levels can be very high (Vanderpool, 1984).

Identifying realistic care goals is vital, as is the need to acknowledge openly that the potential for change in some individuals may be severely limited. The care team needs also to be aware that 'difficulties' expressed by certain patients may be specific to certain members. Decision-making is rarely easy. Difficult decisions, of an ethical nature, concerning disturbed patients, can be highly stressful (Melia, 1988). Nurses who deliver poor quality patient care, or who abuse patients, often do so as a function of chronic stress.

Organization

Many nurses blame themselves when they find it difficult to cope. Stress is seen as a *personal* problem which should be solved by the individual nurse (Hingley and Harris, 1986). Others have argued, however, that organizational factors are often involved and must be part of any solution. Shift-work has been a popular target in stress research. Night duty, in particular, with its disruption of circadian rhythms, has long been recognized as a potential stress area. Afternoon shifts may, however, be more stressful, where a great number of tasks are involved and engagement with relatives and other visitors is required. The nurse's efficiency and productivity may be lowest here, with the corresponding experience of stress at its highest (Coffey, Skipper and Jung, 1988). Where both nurse and spouse pursue full careers, additional pressure may exist (Cooper, 1981). Where both partners are nurses, special stresses appear to be present (Cronin-Stubbs and Brophy, 1984). In a similar vein, domestic responsibilities may conflict with professional responsibilities, causing 'role-strain'; this can also happen when too many demands are made on an individual or when people suddenly change their expectations (Langer and Michael, 1963). Newly-promoted nurses, or those who are elected to professional committees or working parties, may be especially prone to such stress.

Effective 'personnel management' involves structuring a supportive, facilitative environment. Organizational stress is a broad concept. Inadequate support services, poor staff development or continuing education programmes, weak leadership or deficient communications, can all have negative effects. The assumption that such stress is a necessary part of the working environment needs to be *seriously* challenged.

Stress effects

These few examples emphasize a common set of stressors: the nurse's expectations related to her role as a 'carer' and her feelings about whether or not they are realized; the technical demands of care delivery and their effect on the nurse's relationship with the patient; the various issues concerning the organization of care, involving support from the wider health environment. These issues are in no way exclusive to the hospital setting. Health visitors, for example, have identified workload, difficult cases, and feelings of inadequacy, isolation and guilt, as accounting for more than one-half of the stresses felt by this group (West and Savage, 1988).

Nurse Managers, educationalists and researchers, are all potential stress victims. The stressors may be different but with similar effects.

ON BECOMING A NURSE

The world of the student nurse is no less stressful. The demands of the classroom and examination system pose similar problems for all students. Transferring skills and knowledge to a clinical setting carries additional problems. Educational research suggests that many students are unprepared for the 'reality shock' encountered in the clinical environment (Pugh, 1986). This may be one reason for nurses leaving the profession. The stress felt by students may be related to the preparation given to help them deal with the patient as a human being. The technical understanding of specific procedures is useless without the ability to meet the psychological needs of the patient, especially where the patient is distressed.

There is a need to temper idealistic notions of care with awareness of the reality of the patient's condition, or the services available to support him. Educators need also to be aware of potential conflict between their teaching of what should be done and the everyday clinical reality. Students may be encouraged to adopt values which conflict with the behaviour they are 'allowed' to show in the clinical setting (Rickard, 1981). Festinger's (1957) theory of cognitive dissonance is often used to interpret such conflicts. Where people experience conflict between specific cognitions, either information, beliefs, values or attitudes, then a state of tension develops. The person tries to balance all she knows about herself, her behaviour and environment. Students who are given the 'information' that all patients can be helped to recover and who then work with clinicians who suggest that some patients cannot be helped will experience cognitive dissonance. The nurse is torn between two widely differing viewpoints. As a result, she is likely to switch off to the viewpoint which differs most from her own views, or beliefs, in order to maintain her cognitive balance or consonance. Students who become anxious or frustrated in this way may rationalize their sense of failure of helplessness by becoming cynical. As nurses are invited to embrace 'holistic' care, the question is asked how many are prepared for such a demanding role. Some would say that merely proposing such lofty ideals may lay the foundation for 'burnout' (Farabaugh, 1984).

Stress and 'burnout'

The stressful environment stimulates a range of physical and emotional problems. The job may cause the nurse to feel fatigued, at times anxious, occasionally dissatisfied, ultimately sensing a loss of commitment. The nurse may feel moody, or guilty, with lapses of concentration or forgetfulness, at the same time being sensitive to minor physiological changes (after Niehouse, 1981). Most nurses find that two days off, or a holiday, restores their equilibrium. Where stress is maintained at a high level, however, either through environmental demands or high personal expectations, 'burnout' is likely. Fatigue becomes more chronic, the nurse feels unfulfilled and unrecognized, expressing cynical views about a job which is inherently 'boring'. She may become detached, denying any disturbing feelings, but appearing impatient, irritable or depressed to others. She may be so forgetful as to appear disorientated and is likely to express a variety of psychosomatic complaints. Although this process develops steadily across time, burnout is often conveniently described in four stages: (a) enthusiasm, often an unrealistic or fervent nature, is shown early in her career; (b) stagnation develops as goals are not realized and job satisfaction is impaired; (c) frustration, as she recognizes that changes need to be made but she has not the power to effect them, leading to (d) withdrawal as she 'opts out' of responsibilities, or denies feelings, often with accompanying depression or apathy. Although action can be taken at any stage, prevention is better than cure. A task-centred approach to the prevention of burnout is reflected in the organizational acronym T-A-S-C which reflects many of the organizational factors noted above (Squires and Livesley, 1984).

Tell employee standards and goals
Ask employee for suggestions
Set realistic objectives
Check progress and give feedback.

STRESS MANAGEMENT

Effective management of stress begins with its recognition (Bond, 1986). Ideally, the nurse should try to be 'self-aware' in the broadest sense: acknowledging, clarifying and bringing to full consciousness the thoughts, feelings, beliefs and attitudes which are all part of the everyday experience. Practical stress management involves recognizing the causes and effects of stress: increases in tension, loss of concentration, indecisiveness, anxiety and worry. If the 'trigger' can be identified steps may be taken to adjust the stressor at source. Where this is less clear, it may be necessary to settle for learning new ways of coping with stress. There appear to be four main implications of stress in nursing:

- *Self management*: Learn how to manage one's-self more effectively, to reduce the debilitating effects of stress where it is a necessary part of the job. Acquiring skills in self-relaxation of meditation, practising yoga or participating in a regular, controlled exercise programme, managing free time, modifying diet, programming more rest, or generally reducing the 'pace' of life outwith work by negotiating with family and friends, all can have beneficial effects. Any form of easy 'action' — swimming, walking, relaxation exercises — will be more helpful than sitting in front of the television. Selection of the appropriate tactic is important and involves understanding the kind of stress experienced.
- *Environmental modification*: In collaboration with the managers, to become more aware of the negative effects of the working environment. Consideration needs to be given to the care needs of the patient population, staffing resources, the organization of care, including shift-systems, allocation of duties, support within and outwith the care team, in an effort to identify actual or potential problem areas.
- *Realistic goal-setting*: A staff development, or personnel appraisal programme can be used to evaluate the current relationship to the job. What are the nurse's attitudes towards nursing in general? What are the expectations of the present post, patients and of the nurse herself as the

'carer'? This appraisal can serve as the basis for realistic goal-setting, helping the nurse to become clearer as to the real potential for care in her present setting.

- *Counselling*: The three measures above all require some form of 'counselling', even where the nurse is largely counselling herself. Where stress is persistent or acute, more formal psychological support may be indicated. This is best organized on an individual basis. Sharing the problem in a group, under skilled leadership, may be the best way to reach a solution where more general problems exist (Swaffield, 1988; Trevelyan, 1988).

RULES FOR POSITIVE STRESS MANAGEMENT

1. *Taking it easy*   There is a limit to how much the body can take. Make sure that it is getting enough rest, even if it means turning down social invitations. Programme gentle exercise and other forms of active relaxation into free time. 'Real breaks' must not be skimped; day off and holidays must be used to get different kinds of stimulation. The body will be grateful for these considerations.

2. *Being good to one's-self*   Take care over what is eaten. Experiment with the diet; does cutting out specific foodstuffs make any difference? Is the body's coping potential lowered through too much caffeine, nicotine, alcohol, etc.? Think about the kind of things that can be done to boost flagging spirits.

3. *Ducking for cover*   Sometimes withdrawal is the only solution when stress is sustained or very acute. Is it really true that only *the individual* can deal with a stressful situation? Is it necessary to be 'available' at any time, responding to all demands, baling out everyone in distress? Staying in the firing line too long and the risk of getting shot.

4. *Getting one's-self together*   Much stress can be traced to bad organization. Is the daily work schedule planned? Are negotiations made and colleagues and patients told what your plan is? Are difficult or dull tasks, like paperwork or studying, tackled in short bursts rather than marathon trials? If others are really asking too much, they must be told. Only then can a realistic schedule be negotiated. Stressors must be discovered and must be avoided as much as possible. There are no medals for gallantry in the field of stress.

5. *Laughing*   Not all stressful situations have their funny side, but some do. Let others point out what a fool one is, if it cannot be seen by one's-self. Then laugh at one's foibles and failings. It may be better than crying, screaming or protesting. Outside of work, look for laughs; it is probably the best therapy and certainly is the cheapest. Much stress comes from taking one's-self and others too seriously. The person who does not behave like a fool (regularly) has not yet been born.

6. *Sharing all of one's-self* Are friends and colleagues expected to help solve problems and cope with bad experiences? If not, why not? Talk to others. Find out that you are not alone. Find out that not only can they help you but they may be grateful for your support and reassurance. Friends and colleagues will value you more if you quit pretending that you have no problems. A problem is only peculiar to you if you hide it from everyone.

7. *Do not step out of line* Beware of the temptation to believe that you can always influence other people, or take over some of their responsibilities. Do you get angry when other people 'won't co-operate', or 'keep making mistakes'? Are you tempted to make decisions for patients or colleagues on the assumption that they 'are not capable'? Do you try to 'fill in' or substitute for other people's family or friends? Do not stop trying to negotiate with, or even to influence, people. Do not forget that others, like yourself, have the final say. All of us stand alone. We cannot be of real help to others until we recognize this.

8. *Aim* If you never try, you can never win. But are you trying to attain the impossible? Are you aiming to fail? Find out what you *can* do, and get on with it. Forget about what you think you *should* be doing. If you need to acquire new skills or knowledge, take some training. Avoid punishing yourself because you cannot be all things to all men. Make the most of what you are.

9. *Thinking of a number and doubling it* If time was not important, stress would be greatly reduced. Everything takes time and often there is just not enough of it. Getting the job done is the important thing, not how long it takes. Run when problems are life-threatening. At all other times, walk. Think about the time allowed to study for examinations, getting to know a patient, working out a duty rota, or getting to work. Is this adequate or just another added pressure? More time should be allowed than is necessary then the excess time can be worried about. Why the need to hurry? It will always be finished at the end.

10. *Passing it on* Being a professional means knowing what is expected of one, and trying to honour one's responsibilities. Care should be taken not to give one's-self responsibilities or to harbour unrealistic expectations. Asking colleagues and patients what are their expectations of one can be very enlightening. It may be found that they are happy to settle for a little, delivered often. Beware of acting as if one is the only person who can solve the patient's problems.

ANTICIPATION AND REACTION

Most people wait until long after a crisis before seeking help. Vague fears about being seen as a 'complainer' or 'inadequate' lead people to wage a long struggle with their difficulty until forced to give up. By this stage, the problem looms large and the person feels quite hopeless. This is as true of people who are patients as it is for those who are paid careers. Indeed, nurses have a very bad record of helping one another and an even worse record of owning up to fairly normal human failings. The idea that angels can develop wing strain seems never to have occurred to some nurses.

The effect of stress on individuals has been experienced by most of us, more often than we might care to admit. It leads to smoking, eating and drinking more, promoting impulsive, often anti-social behaviour, sometimes causing all manner of aches and pains, the physical sensation of anxiety and agitation, often accompanied by feelings of lethargy, boredom, distractability or apathy. Chronic stress can disrupt family life and other relationships, can contribute to hypertension, heart disease, ulcers and general debility, and various forms of psychological disorder which, in severe cases, can end in suicide. Such recognition of the effects of stress is realistic rather than alarmist. Individual nurses who are concerned to develop their careers cannot afford to ignore stress, which will be part of their professional reality. It leads to inefficient and ineffective service delivery and often seriously damages the health and well-being of patients (Health Education Authority, 1988).

CONCLUSION

Some of the references cited in this chapter show that whole texts can be devoted to the causes of stress in human services, far less their resolution. Many issues highlighted here are reflected in Chapter 20. The development of one's personal capacity to deal with stress can be helped by the social milieu of colleagues and other advisers who offer support. There is much, however, that can be done personally. Ideally, nurses need to anticipate stress in their professional lives, preparing to deal with it realistically, through the best means at their disposal. Stress cannot be managed, however, merely by gritting one's teeth. More thought needs to be given to how we might cope with stress. Stress often has to reach chronic levels before any 'reaction' is taken.

Nurses might do well to model themselves on professional athletes, who treat their bodies and their minds as the vital 'tools' of their trade. Athletes who injure themselves through heroic foolishness, or who function way below par due to inadequate or excessive training, command little sympathy: 'they should know better'. The psychological and physical health of the nurse is vital to the practice of her profession. We need to encourage awareness of the 'pathological' nature of many aspects of our working environment, and of the potential for self-damage within each of us. We need to help one another to find alternative ways of coping with stress and, through sharing, of unloading some of the burden we carry. Above all, we need to treat ourselves with the highest respect.

The hypothetical stress model, which opened this chapter, suggested that stress was highest when the ability to respond to situations, or even belief in that ability, was lowest. The resolution of such stress is, in principle, simple: reduce the gap to more reasonable proportions. Given that stress within nursing is 'occupational', the problem becomes one of professional development. Greater knowledge and skill will reduce the gap between their personal 'resources' and 'demands'. Professional stress is a clear index of the need for professional development. If nurses 'suffer' distress, the quality of care will, ultimately, suffer.

REFERENCES

Astbury, C. (1986) Stress on operating days. *Nursing Times*, **82**(33), 55–6.

Athlin, E. and Norberg, A. (1987) Caregiver's attitudes to and interpretations of the behaviour of severely demented patients during feeding in a patient assignment care system. *International Journal of Nursing Studies*, **24**(2), 145–53.

Bond, M. (1986). *Stress and Self-awareness; a Guide for Nurses*, Heinemann, London.

Coffey, L., Skipper, K. and Jung, F. (1988) Nurses and shiftwork: effects on job performance and job-related stress. *Journal of Advanced Nursing*, **13**, 245–54.

Cooper, C.L. (1981) *Executive Families under Stress*, Englewood Cliffs, N.J., Prentice-Hall.

Cronin-Stubbs, D. and Brophy, E.B. (1984) Burn-out: Can social support save the psychiatric nurse? *Journal of Psychosocial Nursing and Mental Health Services*, **23**, 8–13.

Donovan, M.I. (1981) Stress at work: Cancer nurses report. *Oncology Nursing Forum*, **8**(2), 22–5.

Farabaugh, N. (1984) Do nurse educators promote burnout? *International Nursing Review*, **31**(2), 47–52.

Festinger, L. (1957) *A Theory of Cognitive Dissonance*, Stanford, Calif., Stanford University Press.

Firth, H., McKeown, P., McIntee, J. and Britton, P. (1987) Professional depression, 'burnout' and personality in longstay nursing. *International Journal of Nursing Studies*, **24**(3), 227–37.

Fromant, P. (1988) Helping each other. *Nursing Times*, **84**(36), 30–1.

Gardner, E.R. and Hall, R.C.W. (1981) The professional stress syndrome. *Psychosomatics*, **22**(8), 672.

Hague, C. (1987) Caring can damage your health. *Intensive Care Nursing*, **8**(2), 22–5.

Hare, J., Pratt, C.C. and Andrews, D. (1988) Predictors of burnout in professional nurses working in hospitals and nursing homes. *International Journal of Nursing Studies*, **25**(2), 105–15.

Health Education Authority (1988) *Stress in the Public Sector*, Health Education Authority, London.

Hingley, P. and Harris, P. (1986) Burnout at senior level. *Nursing Times*, **82**(31), 28–9.

Huckaby, L.M.D. and Jagla, B. (1979) Nurses' stress factors in the intensive care unit. *Journal of Nursing Administration*, **9**(2), 21–6.

Jones, G.J., Janman, K., Payne, R.L. and Rick, J.T. (1987) Some determinants of stress in psychiatric nursing. *International Journal of Nursing Studies*, **24**(2), 129–44.

Langer, T.S. and Michael, S.T. (1963) *Life Stress and Mental Health*, Collier Macmillan, London.

Lazarus, R. and Folkman, S. (1984) *Stress, Appraisal and Coping*, Springer Publishing, New York.

Melia, K. (1988) To tell or not to tell? *Nursing Times*, **84**(30), 37–9.

Niehouse, O.L. (1981) 'Burnout': A real threat to human resources managers. *Personnel* (USA), **58**(5), 25–32.

Parkes, C.M. (1972) *Bereavement: Studies of Grief in Adult Life*, Penguin, Harmondsworth.

Pot-Mees, C. (1987) Beating the burn-out. *Nursing Times*, **83**(30), 33–5.

Pryser, P. (1984) Existential impact of professional exposure to life-threatening or terminal illness. *Bulletin of the Nenninger Clinic*, **48**, 357–67.

Pugh, J. (1986) Avoiding stress. *Senior Nurse*, **4**(5), 6–7.

Rickard, T. (1981) Cognitive dissonance: The learner's experience. *British Journal of Psychiatric Nursing*, **1**, 6–7.

Selye, H. (1956) *The Stress of Life*, McGraw-Hill, New York.

Squires, A. and Livesley, B. (1984) Beware of burn-out. *Physiotherapy*, **70**(6), 235–8.

Swaffield, L. (1988) Sharing the load. *Nursing Times*, **84**(36), 24–5.

Trevelyan, J. (1988) CHAT: For nurses in adversity. *Nursing Times*, **84**(36), 27–8.

Vanderpool, J.P. (1984) Stressful patient relationships and the difficult patient, *Rehabilitation Psychology: A Comprehensive Textbook* (ed. P.N. Krueger) Aspen, Rockville, Maryland.

West, M. and Savage, Y. (1988) Visitations of distress. *Nursing Times*, **84**(31), 43–4.

Chapter 5

Legal issues relating to nursing

JOHN TINGLE

There are legal implications attached to every nursing activity from the making a cup of tea for the patient, to the application of plaster-of-Paris. Today's nurse practices in a much more legalistic working environment than previously. A number of factors are attributable for this including:

1. A new 'patient consumerism' is evident;
2. Patients are more aware of their rights and appear less deferential;
3. Record court damages of over £1 million for medical negligence injuries have been awarded bringing intense publicity to medical negligence issues;
4. The number of successful medical negligence claims against doctors has risen. Subsequently doctors' subscriptions to their defence societies showed in 1988 an 87% increase;
5. Chronic understaffing.

All these factors point to an increasingly litigious health care working environment. The nurse must therefore, as a matter of practical necessity, become aware of the law, the system which has the final say when things go wrong. Lawyers and legislators work from an old established legal presumption, ignorance of the law is no defence. We are all presumed to know the law and cannot say we do not, should legal action result.

Concepts such as 'extended role', 'primary nursing', 'nursing practitioners' and 'patient advocacy' are currently extending the frontiers of nursing. Nurses are having to take on more responsibilities and many forget that this leads to increased legal accountability.

This chapter discusses, primarily, how aspects of English civil law affect the nurse in her everyday working relationships with patients and doctors. The following chapter discusses the nurse's legal relationship with her employer. The law applied in this chapter is the law of England and Wales (termed 'English Law') though many of the principles discussed will have application throughout the United Kingdom and in other countries.

THE NATURE OF ENGLISH LAW

The English legal system is adversarial in nature which means that a court trial takes the form of a contest between opposing sides. In civil law, the bringer of the action, the plaintiff must prove his case on the balance of probabilities to the satisfaction of the court, while in criminal law the prosecution must prove the case beyond any reasonable doubt to the jury's satisfaction.

English law has a tangibility, reports of important judicial decisions are commercially published. English law falls into two basic types: Common law and Statute law. The common law is the law made by the judges when they decide cases. Statute law, also known as legislation is that which has been made by parliament. These two sources of law form the bulk of English law.

THE LAW AS IT AFFECTS THE NURSE

A crime can be defined as an offence against society, individuals or the state. The person found guilty of the crime is liable to be punished. The criminal law can be breached where a nurse assaults a patient or where there is theft of hospital property or the commission of drug offences.

Civil law has the main practical affect to the nurse, in particular the law of torts. A tort can be defined as a civil wrong. An action is brought by a Plaintiff against a Defendant in the County Court or High Court. The main torts which can affect the nurse are Negligence, Trespass and Defamation. The Law of Contract is also of increasing affect in private medicine.

There are criminal and civil court structures in England.

NURSING NEGLIGENCE: AN INTRODUCTION

The following is a case study which will highlight certain nursing, legal issues in negligence. Staff Nurse Jones has only recently qualified. She is placed in charge of a surgical ward with a third-year student nurse. It is a busy ward, consultant Smith asks Nurse Jones to take a sample of some blood from patient (A). Nurse Jones does not feel competent to practice venepuncture yet, and understands that this is 'extended role'. She is going to go on a course in a few weeks time. She informs the consultant of her misgivings but he insists strongly that she get on with her job. Reluctantly, Nurse Jones proceeds and causes patient (A) severe bruising to the arm when she attempts to take the blood. On discharge, patient (A) complains to the hospital authorities about Nurse Jones' conduct.

This problem raises a number of very important current issues of nursing concern. Nurse Jones has been placed in a very difficult position by the consultant, a position which is by no means uncommon. The nurse's right to object to the carrying out of tasks which are commonly termed in nursing literature 'extended role' is raised, as is the precise standard of care to be expected.

If the case proceeded to court, the key issue would be the precise standard of care to be expected from Nurse Jones. The consultant's conduct and her manager's conduct would also be analysed. The tort of negligence is the area of law which would be considered by the lawyers and the judge should the matter ever proceed to court.

THE TORT OF NEGLIGENCE

This tort received its modern formulation in the case in *Donoghue* v. *Stevenson (1932) Appeal Cases p. 562*. The plaintiff drank some ginger beer which had been bought for her by a friend in a cafe. The plaintiff alleged that the bottle contained the decomposed remains of a snail and, as a result, suffered gastro-enteritis. The House of Lords ruled in favour of the plaintiff on the preliminary point of whether the facts disclosed a duty of care between the parties. The case was then remitted for trial, though was never finally decided on. One of the parties to the action died and the action lapsed. The case establishes two important principles.

First, product liability, that a manufacturer of products, which are sold in such a form that they are likely to reach the ultimate consumer in the form in which they left the manufacturer with no possibility of intermediate inspection, owes a duty to the consumer to take reasonable care to prevent injury. Second, a broader principle was established, which basically can be said to be that a general duty of care is owed towards anyone who is foreseeable, as likely to be injured by carelessness. There are three elements which must be satisfied before the tort can be established.

1. A duty of care must be owed;
2. The duty of care must be broken;
3. The breach of duty must have caused the damage.

The burden of proving these matters lies on the plaintiff.

Duty: element one

In a nursing context element (1) is easily satisfied. Nurses clearly owe a duty of care towards their patients. Harm is clearly foreseeable. Elements (2) and (3) are more difficult to establish, the breach of the duty of care, and that the breach caused the damage.

Breach: element two

In regard to the problem outlined above involving Staff Nurse Jones, how would the courts assess element (2), the breach of the duty of care? In order to determine this the court would have to assess the standard of care expected by law and whether Staff Nurse Jones fell below this standard.

Past court cases function to provide illustrations of judicial attitude to this type of problem. Statute law is largely silent on the point. The leading case on the standard of care to be expected from doctors is the case of *Bolam* v. *Friern Hospital Management Committee (1957) Vol. 1, Weekly Law Reports.*

In this case the plaintiff (Mr Bolam) was mentally ill, and was advised by a consultant attached to the defendant's hospital to undergo electro-convulsive therapy. The plaintiff sustained fractures during the treatment. No relaxant drugs or manual control (apart from the support of the lower jaw) were used. A male nurse stood on each side of the couch throughout the treatment. Medical opinion was divided on the desirability of using relaxant drugs/manual control and differing views were maintained on whether a patient should be warned about the risk of fracture. Mr Bolam alleged that the failure to warn him of the risk was negligent. The court did not agree, the doctor's conduct accorded with normal medical practice. McNair J. stated in the case the following on the doctor's duty of care: 'A doctor is not guilty of negligence if he has acted in accordance with a practice accepted as proper by a responsible body of medical men skilled in that particular art...putting it the other way round, a doctor is not negligent if he is acting in accordance with such a practice, merely because there is a body of opinion that takes a contrary view. At the same time that does not mean a medical man can obstinately and pig-headedly carry on with some old technique if it has been proved to be contrary to what is really substantially the whole of informed medical opinion. Otherwise you might get men saying "I don't believe in antiseptics. I am going to continue to do my surgery in the way it was done in the eighteenth century". That clearly would be wrong' (p. 122).

An objective issue is being determined, whether the defendant fell below generally accepted standards of conduct. The law requires the nurse to act reasonably, with the ordinary skill of an ordinary nurse in the relevant speciality. If Nurse Jones was taken to court, expert evidence would be called by patient (A) to determine the reasonable standard of nursing care to be expected in the circumstances. Similarly, expert evidence would be brought by Nurse Jones. The judge would then have to decide, from the evidence, the reasonable standard of nursing care and whether in fact Nurse Jones fell below that judicially constructed standard of care. If the judge decides that Nurse Jones's conduct had fallen below reasonably accepted standards she will be found to be negligent. The Bolam case will be cited in court, and will be the main judicial authority relied on by the judge.

Nurses can be negligent through lapses or omissions in their patient care. Nurse managers could equally be negligent if they allow inexperienced staff to occupy key posts in units and perform functions which are beyond their competence or experience. Unsafe systems of work established by hospital authorities which result in injury to staff or patient can result in negligence actions. Negligence can also result through non-communication of information to colleagues about patients' conditions. Nursing process records may not be filled in correctly/sufficiently and a patient's condition may not be fully appreciated. Vousden's (1987) interview with the Health Service Commissioner Anthony Barrowclough revealed the following case:

> But one recent case involving nurses suggests a worrying possibility. It concerned an elderly patient who died avoidably, and one of the commissioner's main criticisms was about the use (or non-use) of the nursing process. The section of the nursing process forms concerning an elderly woman's mobility had not been completed. She was therefore not provided with walking aids or cotsides and subsequently fell three times, sustaining injuries that led to her death (p. 17).

Overwork can also result in negligence, *McCormack* v. *Redpath Brown & Co. (1961) The Times, March 24.* Paull J. held that a failure on the part of a hospital to discover a depressed fracture of the skull and penetration of the bone into the brain tissue was negligent. An overworked casualty doctor assumed, without sufficient grounds, that this was just another of the common cut head cases.

In *Williams* v. *Gwent Area Health Authority June 16, 1982, Current Law Yearbook, 2551, (1983)*, Stephen Brown J. found that a method of lifting patients approved by the hospital was unsafe and negligent, involving extra strain upon the spine. The plaintiff was an Enrolled Nurse and she sustained a back injury when a patient made a sudden movement whilst being moved from bed to a geriatric chair. The method of lifting involved two nurses getting the patient to the side of the bed and then, one on either side, putting an arm under the patient's armpit, with their freehand resting on the bed. The patient was then lifted and turned and placed in the chair at the foot of the bed. The defendants were held 100% responsible for an unsafe system of work. Documents, including statistics which set out the number of reported lifting accidents at the hospital in the area health authority and nationally, showed that there was foreseeable risk of injury to nurses in handling patients.

Negligence through not keeping up to date

Nurses are under a professional duty to keep informed of changes/developments in nursing. The United Kingdom Central Council for Nursing, Midwifery and Health Visiting (1984) Code of Professional Conduct provides in Clause 3 that nurses should: 'Take every reasonable opportunity to maintain and improve professional knowledge and competence.'

The case of *Crawford* v. *Board of Governors of Charing Cross Hospital (1953) The Times, 8th December, 1953* is authority for the proposition that nurses are under a legal duty to keep up to date. The plaintiff Robert Crawford was admitted to the defendant's hospital for an operation to remove his bladder. In theatre, the plaintiff's arm was placed in an extended position at an angle of 90 degrees so that a transfusion could be given. After the operation the plaintiff suffered from brachial palsy in his left arm. Statistics at the time showed that in only approximately one-third of one per cent of such operations did brachial palsy result, and then not permanently. The plaintiff claimed that the anaesthetist Dr Raymond John Clausen had been negligent. The Court found that the defendant had not been negligent and the plaintiff lost his case. The only evidence of negligence was Dr Clausen's failure to read an article which appeared in the *Lancet* in January 1950 six months prior to the operation. The article warned of brachial palsy if the arm was kept in such an extended position. Denning L.J. stated: 'Mishaps often happen without negligence on the part of anybody; the plaintiff here went into the hospital for an operation to save his life, and it has been proved that the hospital exercised all reasonable care. As to the article in the *Lancet*,... it would be putting much too high a burden on a medical man to say that he must read every article in the medical press'. Failure to read one article it was said was not negligence, but disregard of a number of warnings could well be.

This is a common sense decision. An article may appear the following week advocating converse measures. The difficulty in applying Crawford is to determine when knowledge becomes well known and established. A nurse cannot be reasonably expected to keep up with all the new advances and changes, but she must be seen to make some attempt. Her employers should also assist through the provision of post registration education. A health authority which provides little in the way of post registration educational provision is courting disaster and could well be viewed negligent.

Causation: element three

The plaintiff must show that the carelessness of the defendants was the cause of his injury. There must be a causal connection between the act complained of and the injury suffered. The case of *Barnett* v. *Kensington*

Hospital Management Committee (1969) 1 Queens Bench Reports p. 428 illustrates the point.

In this case, a patient presented himself at a casualty department complaining of vomiting. The doctor did not come down to casualty to examine the patient; he was referred to his own doctor and sent away. The patient was in fact suffering from arsenical poisoning and died five hours later. His widow failed to recover any compensation despite the apparent negligence. The evidence was such that diagnostic tests could not have been completed in time and he would have died anyway. There was no link between the breach of duty and the resultant damage. The second and third elements of the tort of negligence, as discussed earlier in the chapter, were not satisfied. Causation was also an issue in the Wilsher litigation to be discussed later.

THE PRINCIPLE OF VICARIOUS LIABILITY

This principle operates in the law of tort to make the employer jointly liable with the employee for any torts committed by the employee. Normally, the plaintiff sues the employer and any damages are paid by the employer regardless of whether the employer was actually at fault. The employer 'stands in' for the employee and assumes responsibility. The injured plaintiff could still sue the nurse directly. Employers who have been sued successfully can lawfully seek an indemnity from their negligent employee to reimburse them for the damages that they have paid out. This employer's right, to the author's knowledge, has not been used against a negligent nurse by a health authority in England and Wales. Trade union membership will normally include insurance cover against such an eventuality.

RES IPSA LOQUITUR (THE FACTS SPEAK FOR THEMSELVES)

It has been stated that in English law the burden of proving fault lies on the plaintiff, the person seeking damages. In medical litigation this can prove a daunting task. The plaintiff must isolate, probably from a number of biological mechanisms, the cause of his injury to the judge's satisfaction. The principle of *res ipsa loquitur* can aid the plaintiff. Where it applies, the defendant must in effect disprove his presumed negligence. If a pair of forceps are left in a patient, or if a doctor cuts off the wrong leg, *res ipsa loquitur* would apply. Dixon (1984) quotes an interesting medical negligence case: 'An enquiry has begun at a hospital in Vienna into how a man, suffering from a broken leg, was mistakenly given a heart pacemaker' (p. 52).

Res ipsa loquitur would certainly apply in that situation.

THE STUDENT NURSE AND THE TORT OF NEGLIGENCE

Nurse training involves the active participation of the student on wards. Student nurses will give injections, administer drugs, all hopefully under supervision. An important legal issue which is unresolved is the legal standard of care to be expected from the student. Do we say the student only has to function as the reasonable student, or do we expect a higher standard of care, particularly where students are occupying key posts in units because of staff shortages. Is there a legal discount for inexperience?

This issue was considered recently in the context of a junior house officer in the case of *Wilsher* v. *Essex Area Health Authority (1986) 3 ALL England Law Reports p. 801.*

In this case, Martin Wilsher, the plaintiff, was born nearly three months premature suffering from various illnesses, including oxygen deficiency. His prospects of survival were considered to be poor. Martin was placed in a special care baby unit. A junior and inexperienced doctor monitoring the oxygen in the plaintiff's bloodstream wrongly inserted a catheter. He mistakenly placed it into a vein rather than an artery. This resulted in venous, rather than arterial blood being monitored and the plaintiff being given excess oxygen. The junior doctor asked the registrar to check the insertion. The registrar failed to notice the error and replaced the catheter the same way himself some hours later, repeating the junior doctor's error. The plaintiff had been supersaturated with oxygen and, it was alleged, that the excess oxygen in his bloodstream had caused an incurable condition of the retina resulting in near blindness.

The Court of Appeal found the registrar negligent and the health authority were held vicariously liable for his negligence. The junior doctor, however, was not found negligent because he had asked the senior doctor to check the work he had done and had therefore discharged his duty. The court decided a number of issues in this case and the judgments are not free from ambiguity. Mustill L. J gave the leading judgment in the case and stated:

> To my mind, it would be a false step to subordinate the legitimate expectation of the patient that he will receive from each person concerned with his care a degree of skill appropriate to the task which he undertakes to an understandable wish to minimize the psychological and financial pressures on hard-pressed young doctors...In a case such as the present, the standard is not just that of the averagely competent and well-informed junior houseman (or whatever the position of the doctor) *but of such a person who fills a post in a unit offering a highly specialized service (p. 813)* (my emphasis).

The duty of care can be seen to be linked to the post a person occupies and not to themselves subjectively. In asking the question 'what standard of care does a student nurse owe'? The answer will be dependant on what she is in fact doing. If a negligent mistake is made when the staff nurse is actually supervising the task, the student would probably be judged from the standpoint of the reasonable student. Responsibility for the incident would then fall to the supervisor. If the student nurse *asks* for confirmation, checking of her work, then under the authority of Wilsher this would protect her from legal liability. The situation appears to change where the student is put in a key post normally occupied by experienced persons because of staff shortages. Here the law would expect her to perform as a normal post holder would. There would be no discount for inexperience in this situation. On a wide interpretation of Wilsher, a student nurse who has placed in, or accepted, temporary charge of an Intensive Therapy Unit/High Dependency Unit would, for the purposes of establishing negligence and breach of duty of care, be judged from the standpoint of an experienced unit staff nurse. She will be presumed to have the relevant experience. Clearly she will not have such relevant experience, and negligence will have been established.

This case also has implications for the deployment of pool or bank nurses. If the nurse is sent to occupy a key post in a unit, and she has not got the relevant experience, and negligence results she will be probably be judged from the standpoint, not as the reasonable bank/pool nurse but as an experienced ITU/HDU staff nurse. She cannot claim inexperience as a defence. In law, just as the learner driver owes the same standard of care as that of a qualified driver, the student nurse, in my example, owes the same standard of care as the qualified nurse. Martin succeeded in the Court of Appeal but the health authority appealed to the House of Lords where the case was eventually sent back for trial on the issue, not of negligence which had been established but on causation. That is, whether or not the negligence actually caused Martin's condition. The House of Lords did not consider the question of the junior doctor's standard of care. See further Tingle (1987a,b; 1988a).

THE EXTENDED ROLE OF THE NURSE AND NEGLIGENCE

Nurses often find that, when they commence their employment, they are expected to undertake a number of duties which are outside the generally accepted and current scope of nursing practice and have not been included in basic training. These duties termed 'Extended Role' have been probably carried out for a number of years as custom and practice. A typical health authority may maintain the following as extended role duties:

Venepuncture (collection only); Application of plaster-of-Paris; Assisting Consultant Radiologist in arteriography or similar techniques; Suturing of minor and superficial wounds (excluding facial); Suturing of perineal tears and episiotomies; Electrocardiograms; Administration of Entonox Analgesia; Lacrimal Duct washouts; Ear Syringing; Addition of Prescribed drugs to i.v. containers; Emergency Defibrillation.

A nurse may also be bound by her contract of employment to perform certain extended role duties. The staff nurse who joins a dialysis unit may find it a condition of her employment that she performs haemodialysis.

The difficulty in this area is the lack of a common definition of the term 'extended role'. Health authorities do not appear to share a uniform view of what nursing duties qualify as extended role. There appears to be no commonality of definition. A nurse may be allowed to practice an extended role activity in one health authority and, on changing jobs, find that she cannot now perform the extended role. There is certainly no national extended role policy. Some health authorities do not maintain written extended role policies, which adds confusion to the issue. The Royal College of Nursing (1978) define extended role as 'tasks outside the routine scope of nursing ' (p. 17). The Department of Health and Social Security (1977) state on extended role: 'The role of the nurse is continually developing as changes in practice and training add new functions to her normal range of duties. Over and above this, however, the clinical nursing role in relation to that of the doctor may be extended in two ways viz. by delegation by the doctor and in response to emergency'.

Extended role here is referenced as being duties outside the normal nursing range. This is a wide definition. A key point made in the circular is that the nurse agrees to undertake the extended role. Nurse Jones in the hypothetical problem posed earlier (p. 49) can refuse to carry out the doctor's instructions. If it was an emergency situation, then depending on the nature of the emergency, the position would change and the nurse would have to respond to the doctor's directions. Clause 4 of the United Kingdom Centre Council for Nursing Midwifery and Health Visiting (1984) Code of Professional Conduct is clear on this point. Each registered nurse . . . shall: 'Acknowledge any limitations of competence and refuse in such cases to accept delegated functions wthout first having received instruction in regard to those functions and having been assessed as competent.'

Nurses have a legal and professional duty to refuse to accept delegated functions which they feel they are not competent to perform.

Health authorities should ensure, as a matter of practical necessity, that extended role policies are formulated, written and communicated to staff. Nurses should also receive instruction in the extended role and the doctor initially testing the nurse should confirm in writing that the nurse has satisfactorily completed the task and is competent to perform it, and that a certificate of competency be issued and a copy kept by the nurse. A nurse who carries out extended role duties is deemed by the law to be competent to carry them out. As Kloss (1988) states, 'If a nurse takes on a doctor's role she will be judged by the standards of the reasonable doctor'. (p. 43).

For extended role in the context of the theatre nurse see Tingle (1988b).

An issue allied to that of extended role is that of nurses being encouraged to become 'patient advocates' and perhaps correcting, elaborating on, a doctor's statement of the risks of a proposed operation to a patient.

THE NURSE AS PATIENT ADVOCATE : LEGAL IMPLICATIONS

A policy of patient advocacy is fraught with legal implications which are not necessarily apparent to the advocates of such a policy (Tingle (1988c) and United Kingdom Central Council for Nursing, Midwifery and Health Visiting (1989) Advisory Document, *Exercising Accountability*). The issue has been neatly articulated by Wells (1986) in discussing the nurse's role and the patient's informed consent to treatment, a key aspect of the nurse patient advocacy role:

> In some cases, lack of informed consent begins on the day of diagnosis when health professionals choose not to be honest. With cancer, the tumor becomes a wart, a mole, a polyp, or any combination of the three. Thus begins a catalogue of deceit, lies and half truths, which may continue until the patient dies, or someone unwittingly tells him the truth. Nurses have a responsibility to protect the rights of those who are unable, for whatever reason, to look after their own interests.

Conversley, Melia (1986) takes this area of patient advocacy to be dangerous territory for the nurse:

> The profession is perhaps in need of a rethink of the whole business of informed consent, and the part which nursing proposes to play in it. In an increasingly litigious society should we not perhaps be wary of getting involved in areas of practice which are clearly the responsibility of doctors? Consent to medical treatment is not an area in which nurses can ever truly be held responsible. It would perhaps be not only prudent but also morally sound to recognize this fact and leave doctor's business to doctors' (p. 27).

These are two useful views which convey competing perspectives in this debate. The legal perspective to the debate is the real possibility of a nurse being sued for giving negligent information to a patient about the proposed risks of a course of treatment. Presently, it is the doctor's duty to obtain patient consent to treatment and it is the doctor who can be sued if that consent has not been properly obtained. The nursing role is one of giving factual explanations and reassurance. Patients have sued doctors in negligence, in recent cases, for failing to give sufficient information about proposed courses of treatment, failing to warn about material risks which subsequently become manifest.

Health authorities may take the view that a nurse, who adopts a doctor's role and gives a patient detailed information about risks and effects of a proposed course of medical treatment, is not acting within the course of her employment. They can then maintain that they are not vicariously liable for her actions, if she is subsequently sued by the patient for negligence.

The picture is not complete without a few words of how patients who have established negligence are compensated for the things that have gone wrong. The assessment of damages system is by no means a scientific or exact process. It is a very difficult task for a judge to quantify in monetary terms the value of a lost limb, sense and faculty.

THE PRINCIPLE OF FULL COMPENSATION

Our courts operate from the premise of awarding *full* compensation to the victim for his injuries. Compensation is based on the plaintiff's individual personal circumstances. Lord Scarman in *Lim* v. *Camden and Islington Area Health Authority (1980) Appeal Cases p. 174* summarized the courts' philosophy to personal injury compensation awards:

> The award is final; it is not susceptible to review as the future unfolds, substituting fact for estimate. Knowledge of the future being denied mankind, so much of the award as is attributed to future loss and suffering — in many cases the major part of the award — will almost surely be wrong. There is really only one certainty: the future will provide the award to be either too high or too low (p. 183).

Courts have regard to past cases when they assess the plaintiff's non-financial loss, working within certain parameters or brackets. A tariff system operates in an attempt to maintain some consistency of approach.

The system of personal injury compensation in English law has been criticized in recent years. It has been argued that the system is expensive and slow.

A number of reforms have been suggested. The British Medical Association have advocated on a number of occasions the creation of a no fault based compensation system for medical accidents. Under such a scheme the plaintiff would not have to prove fault in an adversarial setting. Such schemes operate in New Zealand and Sweden. The schemes have advantages and disadvantages. Causation may still be an issue and an effective mechanism of medical accountability may be lost in the much more inquisitorial setting of a no fault based system. Doctors would not be subject to court appearances and to this extent the deterrent feature of our present fault based system would be lost. The publicity given to medical negligence cases also provides an educative function to the medical and nursing professions. Reforms are being made to English personal injury litigation procedure. It is now much easier for the patient's advisers to obtain medical reports and evidence. If suitably reformed, our present system can better serve the public interest. The short-term reform options proposed by Ham *et al.* (1988) would provide the necessary refinements to effect a more just compensation system. Their proposals, amongst others' involve:

> ...developing a system to enable health authorities to pool their risks in order to cope with a larger number of successful claims...developing arrangements for medical audit by requiring doctors to demonstrate that they routinely review the quality of their work and by introducing procedures for the reporting of surgical and other incidents on a confidential basis...extending and simplifying disciplinary procedures against doctors.

This chapter has hopefully introduced some of the main nursing, legal issues.

Other nursing, legal issues exist, for example defamation and trespass. The nurse who writes malicious untruths about patients or colleagues in a reference or confidential report could be liable under this tort. Trespass in the form of false imprisonment *may* occur where a nurse locks an elderly patient who has been wandering around the hospital in a room for his own safety, and the elderly patient is not mentally ill. Other 'grey' legal areas here are the use of mechanical or other restraints which can be used for nursing convenience on a care of the elderly ward, e.g. chairs with fixed trays, cot sides, etc.

The important point is that nurses become, as a matter of practical necessity, aware of the legal issues which affect them in their work. Further, they should have regard to ethical, moral issues which can be seen to underpin the law. Ethical concepts such as accountability, responsibility, autonomy, justice are key terms which nurses should be encouraged to discuss. The development of ethical legal perspectives functions to concentrate the mind on safe practices and benefits both the nurse and the patient.

Nurses throughout their careers will inevitably encounter the law. An understanding and an appreciation of law in the early stages of their careers will also be beneficial in that potential legal problems can be perceived and expensive litigation avoided. A study of law can also develop confidence and thus enhances nursing status and personal and professional autonomy.

REFERENCES

Department of Health and Social Security (1977) Health Circular HC(77)22. *The Extended Role of the Clinical Nurse—Legal Implications & Training Requirements*, Department of Health and Social Security, London.
Dixon E. (1984) *The Theatre Nurse and the Law*, Croom Helm, Beckenham, Kent.

Ham, C., Dingwall, R., Fenn, P. and Harris D. (1988) *Medical Negligence, Briefing Paper No. 6*, Kings Fund Institute, London and Centre for Socio-Legal Studies, Oxford.

Kloss, D. (1988) Demarcation in medical practice: the extended role of the nurse. *Professional Negligence*, **4**(2), 41–7.

Melia, K. (1986) Dangerous territory. *Nursing Times*, **82**(21), 27.

Royal College of Nursing (1978) *The Duties and Position of the Nurse*, Royal College of Nursing, London.

Tingle, J.H. (1987a) Nurses and the law, *Senior Nurse*, **7**(5), 43–4.

Tingle, J.H. (1987b) Negligence and the law, *Senior Nurse*, **7**(6), 15–16.

Tingle, J.H. (1988a) Negligence and the Wilsher, *Solicitors' Journal*, **132**(25), 910–11.

Tingle, J.H. (1988b) How law is increasingly affecting the practice of nursing. *NAT News. The British Journal of Theatre Nursing*, **25**(10), 25–6.

Tingle, J.H. (1988c) Patient advocacy: the importance of recognising legal implications. *Nursing Times*, Letter, **84**(44), 14.

United Kingdom Central Council for Nursing, Midwifery and Health Visiting (1984) *Code of Professional Conduct for the Nurse, Midwife, and Health Visitor*, 2nd edn, London.

United Kingdom Central Council for Nursing, Midwifery and Health Visiting (1989) *Advisory Document, Exercising Accountability*, London.

Vousden, M. (1987) When the care collapses. *Nursing Times*, **83**(8), 16–7.

Wells, R.J. (1986) The great conspiracy. *Nursing Times*, **82**(21), 22–5.

FURTHER READING

Age Concern (1986) *The Law and Vulnerable Elderly People*, Age Concern, Mitcham, Surrey.

Brazier, M. (1987) *Medicine Patients and the Law*, Penguin, Harmondsworth.

Mason, J.K. and McCall Smith, R.A. (1987) *Law and Medical Ethics*, 2nd edn, Butterworths, London.

Medical Defence Union (1986) *Consent to Treatment*, Medical Defence Union, London.

Rumbold, G. (1986) *Ethics in Nursing Practice*, Baillière Tindall, Eastbourne.

Young, A. (1989) *Legal Problems in Nursing Practice*, 2nd edn, Harper and Row, London.

Chapter 6

Employment law and professional discipline

JOHN HODGSON

GENERAL EMPLOYMENT LAW

The contract of employment

This is only a brief introduction; for more information see Selwyn (1988). Employment is based on contract or agreement, although many rights and obligations arise from statute such as maternity pay, others from collective bargaining such as the Whitley Agreement, others are imposed by the employer such as the salary scales of the Review Body. A contract of employment needs no formalities, and can be oral, written or both. New employees are entitled within 13 weeks to a written statement of their principal terms and conditions. This often incorporates other documents (for instance, a pay scale) by reference.

Obligations of the parties

Both parties must honour their express obligations; there are also implied obligations. Employers must treat employees with reasonable courtesy and consideration, and have reasonable regard to their personal circumstances. Employees must operate professionally, flexibly and reasonably in furthering the employer's operations.

TERMINATION OF EMPLOYMENT

Contract law

Employment results from an agreement and can be terminated by the parties. It can be for a fixed period. If it is indefinite it can be ended by giving suitable notice. In either case it can end earlier by mutual agreement. A party aggrieved at the termination of the contract has no redress, because there has been no breach of contract and therefore nothing for the courts to remedy. The main problems are:

- Disputes over length of notice where there is no express agreement. The court must fix a reasonable period of notice by reference to general practice.
- Unilateral premature termination. This is a breach of contract, and the guilty party is liable in damages. Employers can rarely prove any actual loss when an employee leaves without notice. Employees can claim the financial loss directly resulting from the premature termination (which means loss of earnings for the lost notice period). This is a claim for wrongful dismissal. The court cannot order reinstatement or give compensation for wider categories of loss (for instance reputation or professional development). A premature dismissal is not wrongful if it is a response to gross misconduct, which takes many forms, including dishonesty, serious insubordination, sexual impropriety on duty, violence, misuse of drugs or gross negligence in relation to a patient.

Statutory notice

There are now statutory minimum periods of notice, although the contract may specify a longer notice period. Employees must give one week's notice after four weeks' employment, while employers must give one week's notice during the first two years of employment, and thereafter one week's notice for each full year of employment up to a maximum of 12. Employers can still dismiss summarily for gross misconduct.

Continuity of employment

The rules above apply to all employees, irrespective of their length of service. Many statutory rights described later depend on the employee having completed a period of continuous employment either with one employer, or with a series of associated employers.

- Continuous employment means working under a contract of employment normally requiring work for 16 hours per week or more, although employees who work for five years under a contract normally requiring eight hours or more of work per week will be treated retrospectively as having been continuously employed throughout. Sickness, holidays and strikes do not break continuity.
- Associated employers. Two or more employers in the same group of companies, or controlled by the same person are treated as one employer. This does not apply to the constituent parts of the National Health Service, although it does apply to local authorities.

Redundancy

Redundancy is the dismissal of an employee whose services are no longer required. NHS redundancy arrangements are covered by the Whitley Agreement which excludes the general statutory scheme described below.

- An employee is redundant for statutory purposes only when dismissed because the employer is ceasing to carry on business, or his need for employees of that type is ceasing or diminishing; the situation may affect either the whole of the business or the place where the employee is employed. The closure of a private hospital, or a change in the services offered requiring different skills from the nursing staff might produce a redundancy situation.
- Compensation is by way of a statutory redundancy payment calculated by reference to a week's pay, open to those aged 20 to 65 (men) and 60 (women) with a minimum qualifying period of two years' continuous service and for a maximum of 20 years' service.
- A week's pay is based on normal salary, averaged if necessary, with a statutory upper limit.
- There is no redundancy if there is other work available within the employee's job description, or suitable alternative work is offered and unreasonably rejected.

Unfair dismissal

Employees now have, in unfair dismissal, an effective statutory remedy against improper dismissals. A dismissal may be both unfair and wrongful, but there is no necessary connection; an unfair dismissal where proper notice was given will not be wrongful. Cases of unfair dismissal are heard by Industrial Tribunals. The concepts of fairness and unfairness have to be applied in accordance with the words of the statute, and not with general notions of right and wrong.

Entitlement to claim unfair dismissal

- The employee must normally have two years' continuous service at the effective date of termination of the employment.
- The employee must not have passed the normal retiring age for the employment. The contract of employment may specify a normal retiring age; if not any usual practice is followed. Failing that, the age limit will be 65.
- An employee under a fixed term contract for more than a year can formally abandon the right to claim unfair dismissal on non-renewal of the contract.

Dismissal

Three situations count as dismissal. The first is where the employer terminates the employment, with or without notice (a dismissal in everyday language). Whenever the employee is allegedly in breach of contract it is the employer who terminates the contract. An employee who simply absents herself from work will normally be dismissed as and when the employer indicates that the employment is ended. The second is where a fixed term contract expires and is not renewed (unless the employee has waived her rights). The third and most complicated is the situation known as 'constructive dismissal.' This occurs where the employee terminates the contract and could have terminated it without notice as a result of the employer's conduct, in the sense that he has seriously breached the contract of employment, for example by forcing the employee to undertake non-contractual duties, or breach of the duty of respect (managerial inaction in the face of sexual harassment has been held to constitute constructive dismissal). The employee must prove she was dismissed, if this is in dispute. Ordinarily, an employee who has resigned will not be entitled to claim unfair dismissal. Constructive dismissal is an exception to this rule. An employee who, on being told 'Resign or be sacked' decides to resign may prove that this amounts to a dismissal because of duress, but a resignation to forestall disciplinary proceedings which might lead to dismissal will usually be taken at face value.

The reason for the dismissal

Once dismissal is established, the employer most show the reason for dismissal. A dismissal is automatically unfair unless it is for one of the statutory reasons:

- *Capability and qualifications.* There is no protection during the first two years of employment, so problems of competence arising during a probationary period can be resolved without giving rise to a claim.
- *Basic incapacity*; or inability to do the assigned job. For dismissal to be fair it must be shown that appropriate training and support have been given and the employee has been advised that performance is inadequate.
- *Decline in performance.* This may be due to a change in attitude or isolated episodes of negligence meriting warnings. If the negligence is life-threatening, a single instance may justify dismissal because of the consequences of a repetition. A single negligent heavy landing of an airliner justified dismissal of the pilot, and similar reasoning could apply to a nurse in connection with life support systems.
- The employer need only show that he genuinely and reasonably believed the employee to be incompetent or negligent; not that she actually was.

- *Long-term ill-health*; a sick employee cannot do the job. A balance has to be struck between the interests of employer and employee. The expected duration of the illness, the prospects of full recovery and the length of employment are all relevant factors. The nature of the work is also important. The absence of one employee in a group with similar qualifications and experience may not cause any real disruption to the system, and can be tolerated almost indefinitely, while the absence of a key employee may require the speedy engagement of a substitute, and termination of the original employment. It is generally unreasonable to dismiss during a period of contractual paid sick-leave.
- *Qualifications*; cases on missing professional qualifications are rare; they are normally obtained before appointment. A student failing to qualify would justify dismissal. Where some general qualification, such as a driving licence, is necessary for a post (such as a community nurse) then disqualification would justify dismissal. Removal from the register by the UKCC for disciplinary or health reasons would justify dismissal for loss of the relevant qualification.
- *Conduct*. The categories of misconduct are infinite. To justify dismissal the misconduct must make the employee unfitted to continue in employment, that is, it must reflect on her suitability as an employee, and not merely on her general moral character. A nurse getting into debt, or committing adultery may amount to misconduct, but does not affect her suitability as an employee. A dismissal on conduct grounds may be justified by:

  Professional misconduct (which may also be the subject of disciplinary proceedings by the UKCC); misbehaviour in relation to the professional standards of a nurse, such as abuse of drugs, neglect or physical or sexual abuse of patients.
  Industrial misconduct; general misbehaviour at work, such as dishonesty, wilful damage, drunkenness on duty, insubordination and absenteeism.
  Non-work misconduct; misbehaviour away from work which nevertheless reflects on the employee as such, for instance convictions for a sexual offence of employees in charge of children or other vulnerable people.

Where misconduct is disputed, the employer must carry out an appropriate investigation; the person actually dismissing must reasonably believe in the employee's guilt, but it is unnecessary to prove guilt, or await the outcome of any criminal proceedings.

- *Redundancy*. It does not follow that, because there is a redundancy situation, a particular dismissal will be fair. The employee may have been chosen contrary to the provisions of a selection agreement (such as 'Last in, First out'), the redundancy may be a pretext or there may be a failure to consult before the decision to dismiss. In all of these cases, the dismissal may be unfair.

- *Some other substantial reason (SOSR)*. It is impossible to lay down comprehensive guidelines for fair dismissals. SOSR is designed to allow an element of flexibility. SOSR may cover a change in the organization of work falling short of redundancy, or a change in shift or rota arrangements. An employer alleging SOSR must show that dismissal was an appropriate response to the situation.

Fairness of dismissal

Once a permissible reason has been established the Tribunal must decide whether the dismissal was fair or unfair having regard to 'equity and the substantial merits of the case.' This entails a two-stage enquiry; was a proper procedure adopted, and was the decision reasonable.

- Employers should have, and use, a proper disciplinary procedure. Otherwise any dismissal will probably be unfair. These must be a proper investigation and consultation with the employee, but it is the substance rather than the form of the investigation which is important (although this will not justify the employer in disregarding an established contractual procedure).
- The Tribunal must decide whether the decision is one which a reasonable employer could have taken. They are not there to 'second-guess' the employer's actions, and there may be more than one reasonable decision (that is, there is what has been called a 'band of reasonableness').
- The Tribunal may find that, although the dismissal was unfair, the employee has contributed to the dismissal. This contribution may be total where the dismissal is procedurally unfair, but warranted on the merits, or proportional, typically in misconduct cases where the Tribunal considers that dismissal was an over-reaction, but some penalty was called for.
- The employer can rely only on facts known to him at the time of dismissal to support his decision. Anything coming to light later cannot logically be a reason for the dismissal.

Remedies for unfair dismissal

The primary remedy for unfair dismissal is reinstatement in the original post or re-engagement in a similar post. In practice most dismissed employees do not apply for reinstatement, and the Tribunal may rule that reinstatement is impracticable. The usual remedy is therefore monetary compensation. This is subdivided into two elements, a basic award calculated broadly like a redundancy payment, and a compensatory award, designed to recompense for loss of earnings and employment protection rights in a new job. Any unemployment benefit paid is clawed back. The award will be reduced proportionately where the employee contributed to the dismissal. There is a statutory limit. Additional awards may apply in cases where reinstatement has been ordered, but the employer refuses to comply.

SEXUAL DISCRIMINATION (SD)

The law prohibits discrimination against women or men on grounds of sex, and against married persons of either sex on the ground of marital status. The Equal Opportunities Commission is a publicly funded body which both investigates and reports on SD generally, and provides resources to take individual cases to the Industrial Tribunal. The law covers employment, selection for employment, education and training.

Sexual discrimination described

Direct SD occurs where one person is treated less favourably than another overtly on grounds of sex. The motive of the discriminator is irrelevant. The *Nursing Times* (1988) reports a case where a nursing school was held to be guilty of SD in refusing to accept a married woman with children onto a course for which she was otherwise qualified, apparently because her school-age children might interfere with her ability to complete the course, while a male applicant with pre-school children was not even questioned as to their capacity to interfere with his studies; this was direct SD. Indirect SD occurs when a condition is applied across the board, but it can be shown that a significantly smaller proportion of one sex can comply with it, and it is not objectively justifiable. A civil service age limit of 28 for entry to a particular grade was successfully challenged by showing that a significant proportion of potential female candidates for the posts were unable to apply by the correct age because of child-rearing responsibilities. Sexual harassment may be SD if perpetrated by a senior manager, or if management fails to control the actions of junior employees. SD can be hard to prove. Where there are several applicants for a single post, it may be impossible to go behind the ostensible, non-discriminatory reason for rejection. It may be easier to show SD in matters of promotion and in-service training in a large organization where statistical evidence of the treatment of employees is available. The law has to overcome ingrained cultural assumptions about men as breadwinners and the likely interruption of a woman's career by childrearing. Neither of these assumptions is now a lawful basis for decision making, but the message has yet to get through to many managers. It is only lawful to discriminate where there is a genuine occupational requirement for a person of one sex.

Equal pay

European Community law requires that men and women receive 'equal pay for equal work.' The Equal Pay Act 1970 gives effect to this obligation, although in a very convoluted manner. Where men and women are doing like work, or work that has been assessed as equal by a competent, non-discriminatory job evaluation scheme, they must be paid the same. Like work is work that is broadly similar, not necessarily identical. There may of course be an incremental scale and payments for additional qualifications, provided that these are equally available. A job evaluation scheme will be discriminatory if it merely reflects traditional prejudices, overvalues masculine attributes such as physical strength, or undervalues feminine attributes such as dexterity. A woman (or man) can also claim that his/her work is of equal value to work of a different kind performed by one or more men (or women) who work for the same employer.

- The Industrial Tribunal decides whether the work is of equal value. If not, the claim fails.
- The fact that there is also a man doing like work to the woman will not necessarily defeat an equal value claim.
- If the claim succeeds, the term of her contract relating to pay is modified to equate to the man's, even though other terms, such as holiday and sick pay, are more favourable to her already. In other words the terms are taken individually, not as a package.

A claim for equal pay will fail if the difference is due to a genuine material factor (GMF) differentiating the two cases. This may be a non sex-based matter, such as a shift allowance, or London weighting. In equal value cases the definition of a GMF also includes economic factors, so a male comparator's pay can legitimately include a scarcity premium.

RACIAL DISCRIMINATION (RD)

The legislation has much in common with the SD legislation, using many of the same concepts and machinery. The official enforcement agency is the Commission for Racial Equality (CRE).

Types of discrimination

Direct and indirect RD have the same meaning as in SD, although in the context of race. Feinmann (1988), the National Extension College (1988) and the Commission for Racial Equality (1987a) all point to under-representation of ethnic minorities among nurses now in training or recently qualified. It is difficult to assess whether this is due to non-application based on received wisdom about the profession, to inappropriate recruiting procedures, or to racist attitudes on the part of management or senior colleagues.

Scope of discrimination

The Act relates to discrimination on grounds of 'colour, race, nationality or ethnic or national origins.' An ethnic group must have a long shared history and cultural tradition, normally involving a common geographical origin, language, literature, religion and an identity as a separate group within a larger community. RD may occur in appointments, including job advertisements, during employment in relation to terms and conditions (such as assigning all members of a minority group to night shifts, or to unattractive types of work within a general job description) and access to training and promotion, dismissal or any other detriment (which can include racial abuse if perpetrated or condoned by management). It is permissible to discriminate in relation to a post the duties of which involve the provision of personal services promoting the welfare of a defined racial group, where these are most effectively provided by a member of that group, for instance health visiting services specifically aimed at a minority community.

Remedies for discrimination

There is provision for individual and collective remedies. It may be difficult for an individual to allege specific RD and where RD is entrenched and pervasive there may be no individual complainants because they have all been excluded.

- The individual remedy is by complaint to the Industrial Tribunal. There are wide powers to obtain disclosure of the employer's records, which will be particularly useful in cases based on the employer's past record of promotion for minority employees. The Tribunal can make a declaration as to the applicant's rights, an award of compensation (including an amount in respect of injury to feelings) or a recommendation as to steps to be taken to prevent or eliminate discriminatory practices.
- The CRE may carry out investigations into discriminatory practices in any area they consider appropriate. Commission for Racial Equality (1987b) criticized the NHS for poor implementation of anti-discriminatory measures. Their reports are published, and they can issue non-discrimination notices requiring an employer to refrain from future discrimination. If a notice is breached, court proceedings for an injunction can be brought. The publicity accorded to reports and notices is also valuable in influencing the behaviour of employers generally. The CRE also sponsor research which again leads to publications highlighting problems outside the enforcement context. Investigations of both kinds have been carried out in recent years into various aspects of nurse education and deployment in the NHS.

Although it is not mandatory, it is good practice for major employers to develop and put into practice formal racial equality policies.

PREGNANCY AND MATERNITY

Pregnancy

Dismissal for being pregnant is unfair. The usual qualifying period of two years applies. There are exceptions where the woman is unfit to work or cannot lawfully continue working, perhaps because of exposure to chemicals or radiation, and cannot be redeployed to lighter or safer work. It is unfair to use pregnancy as a factor in selection for redundancy, but a pregnant woman has no special rights, and may be selected if she qualifies on length of service and other criteria.

Maternity pay

This is a description of the Statutory Maternity Pay scheme (SMP). There may be a contractual scheme which provides additional benefits. Like Statutory Sick Pay (SSP), the payments are made by the employer. Entitlement depends on length of service 14 weeks prior to the Expected Week of Confinement (EWC).

- With more than two years' continuous service she is entitled to six weeks SMP at 90% of her average pay plus 12 weeks at the lower rate of SMP (the lower rate of SSP).
- With between six and 18 months' continuous service she is entitled to 18 weeks' lower-rate SMP.
- With less continuous service there is no entitlement to SMP but Social Security maternity allowance is payable.

There are detailed notification and administrative rules.

Maternity leave

This again is a description of the statutory scheme and there may be a more favourable contractual scheme, or employer and employee may make a different agreement. The statutory scheme is complex, with detailed requirements as to notice, and time limits. It is easy to lose rights by accident, and any women intending to exercise her rights should ensure she understands the scheme fully and/or takes advice in good time. The scheme provides a period of approximately 40 weeks' maternity leave, by giving a conditional right to return to work thereafter.

- The woman must be employed with two years' continuous service immediately prior to the eleventh week before the EWC. She need not actually be at work then; she may be on sick or annual leave. If a woman actually resigns to take effect before this date, she loses her statutory rights.
- The woman must give three weeks' notice of intended pregnancy absence, that she intends to return to work, and of the EWC. The notice of intention to return is not binding, but should be given to protect the woman's position even if she does not intend to return; her circumstances may alter.
- Seven weeks after the EWC the employer may request the woman to confirm whether she intends to return. She must reply within two weeks.
- Return to work must be within 29 weeks of the actual birth, or earlier at the woman's option, subject to three weeks' notice of the date of return.
- Where the woman has complied with the procedural requirements, but the employer refuses to allow her to return, she is deemed to have been employed up to the date of the refusal and dismissed on that date. The dismissal may be unfair, but special rules apply.
- A woman who fails to comply with the statutory procedure loses her statutory rights, but if her contract of employment continues during her absence she can return to work on reasonable notice. If the employer refuses to allow this, it counts as a dismissal.

NATIONAL HEALTH SERVICE (NHS) CONDITIONS OF SERVICE

The institutional framework

Conditions of service within the NHS are established and altered by a number of bodies at national and local level, each with its own sphere of responsibility, membership and ethos, as described by Borley (1989). Originally the national bodies were the General Whitley Council, covering issues common to all NHS staff and the Nurses and Midwives Whitley Council. The latter was until 1983 the pay negotiating body, but this aspect of its functions is now assigned to the Review Body for Nursing Staff, Midwives, Health Visitors, and Professions Allied to Medicine (the Review Body). In addition to these national bodies, each Health Authority is responsible for establishing detailed local terms and conditions of service. The Review Body receives evidence from the interested parties (Department of Health, management and staff representatives), and presents a report to the Government. Although primarily concerned with salary levels in the light of the economic situation, staffing levels and comparable salaries in other fields, it can range wider than this, and was for instance responsible for the initiation of the recent clinical grading review. The

Secretary of State for Health responds to the report, which may be accepted in whole or part or rejected. Acceptance of the report does not necessarily imply a commitment to fund the award from government resources. The tripartite system whereby the government establishes a national policy and provides funds, but responsibility for budgeting, and for grading the remunerating individual staff lies with the Health Authorities has led to public misunderstanding, particularly of the role of the Secretary of State. The recent White Paper on the Health Service proposes several changes to the negotiating machinery. Self-governing hospitals will negotiate independently. The Review Body is to be encouraged to make recommendations differentiating between nursing specialisms on the basis of supply and demand, so that if theatre nurses, for instance, are in short supply, they can be offered premium rates of pay. The long-term aim is that 'employment packages' are to be locally negotiated.

The contract of employment

The contract of employment is the responsibility of the employing authority. It will incorporate the Terms and Conditions of service of the General Whitley Council and the Nurses and Midwives Whitley Council, and the Review Body's recommendations as brought into effect by the Government, together with any general Policies and Procedures of the employing authority. These documents will be available for inspection. The contract itself will contain personal details and particulars of post held, salary, hours and place of work, leave and notice arrangements; it should, however, be noted that a flexibility clause will usually allow management to override the hours and place of work.

Grievance and disciplinary procedures

The General Whitley Council has a procedure (s32) for the resolution of grievances. The Authority must establish equivalent procedures locally. These will provide for recourse to an immediate manager and then to a more senior manager. Where the grievance concerns Whitley Terms and Conditions the national scheme can then be invoked. The General Whitley Council has also laid down procedural guidelines for disciplinary proceedings (s40), within which each authority is responsible for framing its own rules covering:

- rights of representation
- details of investigation procedures, including powers of suspension
- the forms of disciplinary action available, and the time for which warnings remain effective

- an indication of the way in which different categories of misconduct will usually be treated
- appeal arrangements.

S40 provides rules for the conduct of disciplinary proceedings. There is a mandatory requirement of a warning for a first offence, except where it amounts to gross misconduct. There are detailed requirements as to the officer entitled to dismiss, and provision for a right of appeal to the employing authority. If the position cannot be resolved internally, a dismissed employee can claim unfair dismissal.

PROFESSIONAL DISCIPLINE

The legal framework

The hallmark of a profession is that it is self-regulating. The UKCC exercises this function by statute in relation to nurses, midwives and health visitors. The UKCC makes and enforces the Code of Professional Conduct (CPC), which applies to all practitioners, and the Codes of Practice and Practice Rules for each sector of the profession. The CPC stresses the requirement to promote and safeguard patients' interests and to act responsibly, while the Codes of Practice deal with situations of particular relevance to the group concerned, such as, for midwives, home confinements and registration of births. These are rules of substance, setting out what a particular type of practitioner must and must not do in her practice. The Nurses, Midwives and Health Visitors (Professional Conduct) Rules define the procedure to be followed when there is an allegation of professional misconduct, and the penalties which may be imposed.

The disciplinary procedure

Anyone can make a complaint of professional misconduct, defined in the rules as 'conduct unworthy of a nurse, midwife or health visitor.' All complaints are initially investigated by the relevant national Board, which must notify the practitioner of the allegation and invite a 'written statement or explanation from her.' The Board may simply discontinue its investigation. The rules do not specify when this may be done, but it would cover the case where a complainant refuses to provide further evidence, or a complaint is frivolous. Otherwise, the Board must formally consider the case, although there is no hearing at which the respondent (the subject of the complaint) is present. The Board can reach three conclusions: to refer the case to the Conduct Committee of the UKCC 'with a view to removal from the register'; to refer the case to the UKCC Health Committee because it discloses possible ill-health unfitness rather than misconduct; or to take no further action, if there is inadequate evidence of misconduct, or there is minor misconduct, but no useful purpose would be served by a formal hearing, and they may then (by way of what amounts to an informal reprimand) draw the respondent's attention to the CPC.

The condunct of the hearing

Where a case is referred to the Conduct Committee, the respondent will be notified of the arrangements for the hearing, and of the charge(s) to be considered. She may appear personally, or be represented by a friend, lawyer or official of a professional organization or Trade Union. The case will normally be prosecuted by the UKCC solicitor. The Committee comprises at least three members of the UKCC 'chosen with due regard to the professional fields in which the respondent works or has worked,' to ensure that the respondent is indeed being judged by her peers. The Committee sit with a legal assessor, who advises on matters of law which arise during the hearing. The hearing will normally be in public.

The procedure depends on whether the respondent is present, and if so whether she admits the facts. If she appears and denies the facts the case proceeds like a criminal trial, and the case must be proved beyond reasonable doubt. A charge will be rejected if the facts are not proved. Where the respondent appears and admits the facts, the Committee hears an account of the underlying circumstances from the prosecutor. The respondent may challenge any parts of this. Where the respondent does not appear, but has admitted the facts in writing, the procedure is similar. Where the respondent does not appear and has not admitted the facts, the case must be formally proved.

The Committee then decide whether the facts constitute misconduct, and announce whether they find the respondent guilty of misconduct. If so, they hear evidence as to the previous history of the respondent. This may be general background material, or evidence of earlier findings of misconduct. The respondent may challenge this evidence and make a plea in mitigation.

Powers of the Committee

The Committee must first consider whether to postpone judgment. The respondent may continue in practice. Postponement is a form of probation; at the postponed hearing the Committee will consider reports on the respondent relating to her subsequent conduct and any other relevant evidence. A postponed hearing may be further postponed, in theory indefinitely, but unduly protracted postponement would be unreasonable. The Committee can refer any case which raises issues of ill-health rather than misconduct to the Health Committee. The only final decisions the Committee can make are to take no action on the misconduct (except to draw the respondent's attention to the CPC), or to remove the respondent's name from the register or a part or parts of it, with immediate effect. This decision prevents the practitioner from continuing in practice.

Appeals

There is a right of appeal from a removal from the register to the Courts. The High Court has held in *Hefferen* v. *UKCC The Times, 21st February, 1988* that it 'should not interfere with the decision of the disciplinary committee, experienced as it was, unless it was clear that that decision was wrong.' A decision may also be quashed because of breaches of natural justice (the ground rules developed by the courts to ensure that 'private courts' such as the Conduct Committee operate fairly and reasonably).

The Health Committee

The function of the Health Committee is to establish whether a practitioner should be removed from the register on health grounds. A case may be referred to the Health Committee by a Board or the Conduct Committee during disciplinary proceedings or commenced on health grounds if the Registrar of the UKCC receives information in writing suggesting that the fitness of a practitioner is impaired on health grounds. This is passed to a panel of professional screeners (specially selected practitioners) who consider the evidence. Where there are grounds to take the matter further, the practitioner will be informed and invited to submit to a medical examination. The Health Committee consists of members of the UKCC; one of the medical examiners will be present as an assessor. The proceedings are held in private, but the practitioner is entitled to attend and be represented. The case against the practitioner will be put first; she can then address the Committee and call evidence. Although the proceedings of the Health Committee are formal, its function is not punitive, and so the strict procedures of the Conduct Committee do not apply. The Committee is, however, subject to the control of the courts.

The Committee may make four determinations; to adjourn for fresh evidence; to postpone judgment, setting a date for the postponed hearing and specifying the evidence required at that time; to determine that the practitioner's health is not impaired (when it may, but does not have to, refer a case which came from a disciplinary investigation back to that procedure); to determine that the practitioner's fitness to practise is seriously impaired on health grounds and direct removal from the register.

Restoration to the register

A practitioner who has been removed from the register may apply for restoration. The application will be heard by the Committee which ordered removal, but the procedure is similar in health and disciplinary cases. The Committee hear the facts which led to removal, and anything known of the practitioner's activities in the interim period. The practitioner can address the Committee and call evidence. The practitioner must prove she is fit to resume practice.

The system in operation

The system has not been in operation long. It takes time to get used to a new development of this kind, and it is perhaps not surprising that Pyne (1985) reports that in the early years the majority of misconduct complaints came from employers. In some 45% of cases found proved on misconduct grounds in 1985/6 no action was taken. Vousden (1987) and Morrison (1987) suggest that in many cases the Committee felt that the respondent, although technically at fault, was morally blameless because the problem originated from understaffing, poor supervision or other management failing. In the same period enrolled nurses and those working in mental illness and mental handicap were disproportionately represented. This may reflect poor practice in these areas, or alternatively the high proportion of enrolled nurses in these fields, poor staff ratios and pressure of work. What is clear is that, as Morrison relates, isolated instances of carelessness are being pursued to a hearing. This contrasts with the practice of the General Medical Council which has traditionally differentiated between misconduct and negligence or bad practice, with only the first being subject to disciplinary action. Morrison, as a member of the Conduct Committee, suggests that there is in practice an emphasis on pastoral care which is not expressly part of the functions of the Committee.

TRADE UNIONS

The nature of Trade Unions

Trade Unions are self-regulating voluntary associations of workers, formed primarily to enable members to bargain on terms and conditions of employment with employers. Unions operate benevolent funds, promote training, provide legal assistance with work-related problems, and represent their members, often very effectively, in various proceedings. Unions have traditionally offered negligence insurance cover, and now often offer general insurance and other financial services. With the members' approval, Unions may also pursue political objectives extending beyond the improvement of members' conditions of employment to the organization of society generally. For nursing Unions to enter the debate on the philosophy of health care and the relative roles of the NHS and the private sector is political in this sense. Political activity by Unions in the above sense is a long-standing and legitimate activity, having no necessary connection with party politics. Unions were almost entirely self-governing until the early 1970s. Since then Parliament has intervened to improve their internal democracy, for instance by requiring voting members of the executive to be elected by secret ballot and by requiring a secret ballot to authorize industrial action. These reforms have ensured the right of the individual member to an equal say in Union policy, although many unionists have resented the element of compulsion employed.

Union membership

Workers have the right to join an independent Union and take part in its activities at appropriate times (normally, out of working hours). A dismissal for exercising these rights is unfair, and the normal two-year qualifying period does not apply. A worker also has the right to refuse to join or to resign from a Union. Dismissal for doing so will be automatically unfair, and attracts enhanced compensation.

Recognition of Unions

There is no obligation on an employer to recognize a Union. Employers do so because there are advantages in dealing with bodies which represent a significant proportion of the workforce. Recognition usually carries with it the right to represent individual workers; this policy is followed both in the Whitley Agreement and in the practice of the UKCC.

Collective bargaining

A key function of Unions is negotiating terms and conditions of employment with employers. The original Whitley machinery was a typical example of a formal, permanent collective bargaining set-up. The present scheme is different. Unions make representations to the Review Body, which then makes its recommendation. There is no negotiation. Collective agreements are not legally binding contracts creating enforceable rights and obligations, but where they change the pay or other conditions of a worker, her own individual contract will be amended accordingly, and that contract itself is legally binding.

Industrial action

When negotiations fail, the matters in dispute may be referred to an arbitrator who will determine the dispute in accordance with general notions of fairness and 'industrial justice'. If the arbitrator's decision is binding, that is an end of the matter. Otherwise, the last resort is disruption of the employer's undertaking by industrial action. Although industrial action is a normal way of resolving otherwise intractable disputes, some Unions refuse to take industrial action, or at least to strike, either on principle, or under a 'no-strike' agreement with a particular employer. Unions such as the RCN, which emphasize professional obligations rather than the employment relationship refuse to strike, preferring to rely on public opinion. Industrial action can take a number of forms:

- *Strikes*: the strike is a withdrawal of labour constituting a repudiatory breach of contract by the employee. If the employer accepts the breach and dismisses the employee she cannot claim unfair dismissal unless there is victimization, in that some strikers are not dismissed, or are later reinstated. Employers usually don't dismiss strikers, because of the problems of organizing a replacement workforce, but it has been known. There is a right to strike, in the sense that no court or policeman can force a striker back to work, but the right is exercised at some risk.
- *Refusal to carry out Full Duties*: an employer can insist that an employee carry out all the duties attached to her position. If she refuses to carry out particular duties she can be suspended without pay, or dismissed. Where the employer accepts the situation, a deduction from salary may be made to cover the work not done.
- *Overtime Bans*: if the employee has agreed to work overtime when required, a refusal will be a repudiatory breach of contract, otherwise, an overtime ban is perfectly legitimate.
- *Work to Rule*: may be a breach of an implied (or express) term in the contract to do all that is reasonable to foster the smooth working of the enterprise, or to apply rules flexibly, not pedantically. Sometimes it only involves employees applying rules which exist for their benefit, but which are usually waived. Each case must be judged on its own facts.
- *Work to Grade*: this is a new concept presupposing a conflict between the duties that can be demanded of an employee by reference to the job description and level of seniority indicated by a grading, and the requirements of the actual job the employer requires done. As Finch (1988) observes, the courts have not considered the matter, but in principle it seems that an employee may refuse to do a job appropriate to a higher grade, although it may be unreasonable not to cover temporarily for illness or other emergency. On the other hand, it is wrong to insist upon an unduly narrow definition of the duties appropriate to

a grade, or to refuse to perform tasks traditionally associated with a particular post.

Unions and industrial action

It is normally a tort (a civil wrong, for which damages can be awarded) for A to induce or threaten B to break a contract with C. This covers a Union inducing an employee to break his/her contract with an employer by taking industrial action. *Bona fide* Unions have a statutory immunity from action provided the following conditions are met:

- The industrial action is in pursuance or furtherance of a trade dispute, i.e. a dispute between employer (including a Minister legally responsible for determining pay or conditions, as with the Review Body) and employees over terms and conditions of employment, discipline, employment of any person, allocation of work or Union recognition. Political strikes are excluded.
- Those likely to be involved in the industrial action must have voted to take action in a secret ballot conducted in accordance with rules laid down in the Trade Union Act 1984.
- It must not be secondary action. Immunity extends only to breaches of the contracts of employment of the employees of the employer(s) with whom there is a dispute, and interference with the supply of goods and services to or by him/them and any associated employers, and to lawful picketing.

Where the immunity does not apply, the Union will be liable in damages, and an injunction can be granted to stop it supporting the action. If the injunction is ignored, the Union and its officers will be in contempt of court. The Union's funds are liable to seizure and the officers to imprisonment.

Picketing

Pickets may lawfully attend at or near their own place of work in contemplation or furtherance of a trade dispute with a view to peacefully persuading people to work or not to work and to obtaining or communicating information. Picketing elsewhere or by others is illegal. There are a number of criminal offences associated with excessive or aggressive picketing, from obstruction of the highway or of the police to violent disorder. There is a Code of Practice on picketing which gives guidelines for peaceful picketing.

REHABILITATION OF OFFENDERS

Since the Rehabilitation of Offenders Act 1974 came into force it has for most purposes been the case that those convicted of criminal offences have the right to treat the conviction as spent and themselves as rehabilitated after a specified period. Convictions for which a sentence of more than thirty months imprisonment was imposed are outside the scope of rehabilitation. The period in other cases ranges from ten years for shorter prison sentences to five years for fines and six months for absolute discharges. If there are successive convictions, then if the later one is a serious crime, capable of being tried by the Crown Court in England, or outside the jurisdiction of the inferior courts in Scotland, the earlier conviction will not become spent until the later one is. In most situations a spent conviction can be ignored, and a person with a spent conviction who is asked about previous convictions can ignore it. She cannot be taken to task about it, accused of lying or otherwise penalized or victimized. There are exceptions. This immunity will not apply if questions are put officially in order to assess the suitability of any person for admission to (among others) the profession of nursing or midwifery, to take employment in the field of personal social services or health care, or to carry on a registered nursing home. In relation to these matters, if questions are asked about convictions that would otherwise be spent, they must be answered. If they are not truthfully answered, and the truth later comes out, then sanctions may be imposed, extending to removal from the register or dismissal. The obligation is only to answer the question, not to make full disclosure. If for instance the question excludes, as is often the case, motoring convictions, then these need not be disclosed, whether or not they are spent.

CONCLUSION

Every nurse needs to understand her position as an employee, both in relation to rights and obligations in order to fulfil the obligations and ensure that the rights are respected. Although recourse to formal legal action is a rarity, the law underpins everyday working life. With increasing seniority and management responsibility the nurse will also find herself considering these issues from the perspective of a manager in control of junior staff.

REFERENCES

Borley, D. (1989) Industrial Relations, in *Management and Professional Development for Nurse*, (eds M. Dodwell and J. Lathlean) Harper and Row, London.

Commission for Racial Equality (1987a) *Ethnic Origins of Nurses Applying for and in Training*, Commission for Radical Equality, London.

Commission for Racial Equality (1987b) *Annual Report*. Commission for Racial Equality, London.

Feinmann, J. (1988) The Asian Factor. *Nursing Times*, **84**(43), 18.

Finch, J. (1988) Regrading — the legal aspects. *Nursing Standard*, **3**(13/14), 16–7.

Morrison, I. (1987) Reviewing the evidence. *Nursing Times*, **83**(8), 31–2.

National Extension College (1988) *The Black Nurse: an endangered species*, National Extension College, Cambridge.
Nursing Times (1988) *Nursing Times*, **84**(40), 7.
Pyne, R. (1985) The disciplinary process. *Senior Nurse*, **2**(3), 7–10.
Selwyn, N. (1988) *Law of Employment*, 5th edn, Butterworths, London.
Vousden, M. (1987) Conduct unbecoming. *Nursing Times*, **83**(8), 29–30/33–4.

Chapter 7

Nursing career planning

DESMOND CORMACK

Career planning is a cyclical process which has equal relevance to all stages of a career; it addresses past, present and future stages of development.

Career planning applies equally to those who are seeking promotion, intending to achieve significant changes in career direction, and to those who intend to work in an existing position indefinitely. Collectively and individually, the nursing profession is committed to continuous career planning and development; to be otherwise would cause nursing to be a quasi-profession, and for nurses to be quasi-professionals. The general principles of career planning are the same for all nurses, irrespective of past, present or future career pathways. Because of the general application of basic principles, it is intended that the material in this chapter can be applied by any nurse at any stage of career development. Career planning is not the same as 'job hunting', it is necessary whether or not you are seeking promotion or applying for a job (Jarczewski, 1986). Planning consists of a number of inter-related parts operating on a cyclical basis (Figure 7.1).

ASSESSMENT

Initial training

Irrespective of present career position, planning is firmly based on a thorough assessment of previous professional development. The extent to which initial training requires to be assessed depends on how long ago it took place. If it was recent, within the past two years for example, it requires a detailed assessment. If, for example, it took place a number of years previously, then a more general assessment may be required. In either case, a more or less detailed assessment will form part of an overall review which is undertaken in the light of current circumstances and future plans.

The least that initial training should do is provide an education which produces a reasonably safe and proficient clinician. It is widely re-cognized that it provides a *basis* for future career development. It is also

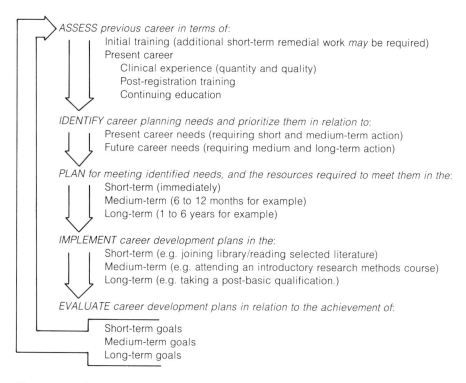

ASSESS *previous career in terms of*:
    Initial training (additional short-term remedial work *may* be required)
    Present career
        Clinical experience (quantity and quality)
        Post-registration training
        Continuing education

IDENTIFY *career planning needs and prioritize them in relation to*:
    Present career needs (requiring short and medium-term action)
    Future career needs (requiring medium and long-term action)

PLAN *for meeting identified needs, and the resources required to meet them in the*:
    Short-term (immediately)
    Medium-term (6 to 12 months for example)
    Long-term (1 to 6 years for example)

IMPLEMENT *career development plans in the*:
    Short-term (e.g. joining library/reading selected literature)
    Medium-term (e.g. attending an introductory research methods course)
    Long-term (e.g. taking a post-basic qualification.)

EVALUATE *career development plans in relation to the achievement of*:
    Short-term goals
    Medium-term goals
    Long-term goals

Figure 7.1 Career planning process.

recognized that initial training requires to be supplemented by additional education once the newly qualified nurse enters the staff nurse grade. Lathlean (1986) identified seven areas in which newly qualified nurses needed to further develop. These were: clinical and managerial knowledge and skills; interpersonal relationships and communication skills; issues relating to autonomy and the capacity for self-direction and analytical thought; personal development such as motivation, awareness of personal needs, strengths and weaknesses; attitudes in relation to current professional philosophy and issues; an understanding of career development issues; and coping with professional stress.

Ioannides (1988) described the setting up and the evaluation of a development programme for newly qualified staff nurses. That programme consisted of six major areas which were: professional issues; nursing research; communications; teaching; nursing management and administration; and legal and personnel issues. Ioannides proposed that the development programme had advantages for the qualified staff nurses, and for the organization in which they worked.

The general recognition that initial training may be inadequate, and the many attempts to 'make good' the shortcomings are the result of a number of aspects of that education. First, the variability of educational programmes, combined with the need to cover a large number of topics, may result in one or more of these being relatively poorly covered. Second, the programme may have been adequate, but the student may have 'struggled' with a topic; passing the examinations although remaining relatively weak in an important subject area. Third, aspects of the training may have been overtaken by events in which new health care problems, clinical techniques, new diseases, and new nursing approaches, have inevitably caused the training to be out of date in a short space of time. The need to assess the adequacy of initial training is emphasized by the notion that recently qualified nurses are probably more ill-equipped and vulnerable than are all other trained nurses for four reasons. First, the recently qualified nurse will be working in a clinical environment for which initial training provided a limited amount of skill and knowledge. Second, she will be experiencing a considerable amount of 'culture shock' and difficulty in adjusting to the transition from student to qualified nurse. Third, she will have relatively little experience of the specialist clinical area. Finally, she will not have had time to fully participate in career development activities.

In addition to possible deficiencies of a clinical nature, it is probable that some of non-clinical aspects of career development have not been fully addressed during initial training. For example, there may have been little exposure to considering job opportunities, applying for a job, being interviewed, contributing to the professional literature, or to the principles of research. Alternatively, these subjects may have been partially addressed. For example, the requirement that students produce a number of essay style reports adds much to the development of those skills required to contribute to the professional literature.

Present career

Clinical experience (quantity)

The quantity of clinical experience relates to the total amount of experience following qualification, and to how that time was distributed between various specialties. At one extreme, all of the time may have been spent in one relatively narrow specialty. At the other extreme, experience may have been gained in a variety of clinical specialties. Although neither quantity of experience is 'best' for all eventualities, each is more or less 'right' for specific types of future career. For example, if it is intended to specialize in the care of the elderly, then spending time in that specialty would be more appropriate than dividing the experience between the care of the elderly, children, intensive care and surgical patients.

Conversely, if one is intending to become a senior nurse manager involved with a variety of specialties, it would be more appropriate to gain a wide clinical experience in these. In the period immediately after qualification, a 'middle of the road' option is best, one which will give a variety of related experiences which will consolidate initial training, and give a preparation for working in either a specialized or more general position. Thus, the decision to over-specialize should probably not be made too early. There can be no doubt that it is essential to undertake a reasonable variety and amount of clinical experience before moving into a largely research, administrative or teaching post. The amount of clinical experience required before moving into these non-clinical positions is usually determined by a combination of personal judgement, and the more formal constraints which are often applied to various non-clinical positions. For example, those who wish to become nurse teachers will require to have had a minimum amount of clinical experience, with some of this time being spent at a specific senior level. Indeed, progress to many non-clinical posts is often only possible by moving through a series of promoted positions, each requiring a minimum amount of clinical experience. Such experience is the foundation upon which all subsequent career development is based. It has a clear relevance to those who spend a life-time working closely with patients, and equal relevance to those who choose to work in non-clinical areas such as teaching, administration or research.

Clinical experience (quality)

The quality of clinical experience is different from the quantity in that the former is governed by the extent to which the experience is positive and of the kind which helps individual career development. The latter is primarily concerned with the amount of time spent in obtaining clinical experience in one or more specialties. The quality of experience is influenced by factors which depend on, and which are partly independent of, the individual. These are: the quality of the staff in the organization, and the quality of the organization itself.

Quality of staff within an organization   It is quite possible for two apparently similar clinical experiences to be very different in terms of quality. This difference results from the varying quality of the staff group. For example, one group might have limited vision and insight. They may take the view that additional personal and collective development is not necessary, and consequently fail to grow and develop within this particular experience. Another group might take a different view and search for opportunities to learn from the experience and try to achieve new understanding and skills. These extreme positions result, in part, from the personality and general make-up of individuals and staff groups. They are also a result of the motivation of the group concerned, and are a consequence of decisions taken by them individually and/or collectively. If the quality of an experience is to be maximized, this can be achieved by working within a milieu, and with a peer group, supportive of the notion of the need for continuing career development.

Quality of the organization   Some organizations have much to offer by virtue of having achieved an organizational and professional excellence, and by having staff who are innovative, challenging and generally rewarding to work with. Although it is possible to find good organizations (employers) with poor quality staff, or poor quality organizations (employers) with high quality staff, the two tend to be mutually exclusive. Thus, good organizations tend to produce (or be the product of) good staff. Poor quality organizations tend to produce (or be a product of) poor staff. The remainder of this section will discuss some key features of an organization which will provide a good quality of experience. The material can be used for the purpose of assessing previous experience; it can also be used to make decisions regarding the type of experience which a prospective employer might provide.

Respect for the employee   The primary obligation of employers is to provide the best possible service to the consumers of their services. In order to achieve this, an employer constructs an organization which will attract high quality staff, and meet the needs of individual employees. A good organization recognizes the personal, occupational and educational needs of those they employ, thereby recruiting high quality staff who will provide a good service. Employees within such an organization are made to feel recognized as individuals who, in addition to having a responsibility to provide high quality care, have career needs identified and met.

Is it innovative?   The extent to which an organization is innovative and dynamic, examining and trying out new ideas and routinely evaluating its own performance requires consideration. There is a need for any complex organization to recognize that it must respond to internal and external needs and developments. Such an organization will provide a rich professional experience in which employee growth will be maximized; it will also considerably improve the quality of care it provides. An important feature of innovative dynamic development is the extent to which individual staff are allowed, and encouraged, to question, challenge and constructively criticize existing procedures, policies and attitudes. This freedom provides a fertile ground for the achievement of a high quality experience (see also Chapter 3).

Staff development   Although the priority for any health care organization is to provide high quality care to its patients, there are a number of ways of utilizing its resources to reach that goal. It is possible, for example, that all resources be used for that immediate purpose (direct health provision), and that none should be made available for the professional development of the staff who deliver that care. Alternatively, the view might be that 'We recognize the need to provide staff development resources. However this would require a shift of resources away from direct patient care.' These views have both a relevance to the short term in which the quality of care is maximized by the allocation of all possible resources to meet that aim.

In considering the medium- and long-term position, many organizations employ strategies which develop and educate professional staff in order to maximize their contribution to care. These opportunities which must use a proportion of available resources (including funds) are a crucial indicator of the quality of past or future work experience. In considering experience quality, ask if staff development opportunities are available, and consider their range and appropriateness.

Very few work environments are at the extreme ends of the continuum in terms of quality, either being wholly adequate or inadequate. The realities and constraints of our professional working lives invariably result in some form of compromise in which we are exposed to varying qualities of experience.

Post-registration training

For some, post-registration training may be necessary (indeed compulsory) prior to entering a particular part of the profession. For example, in order for a nurse to become a registered nurse tutor in the United Kingdom, there is a compulsory requirement to successfully complete a course leading to a qualification in that area. In other instances, a specialized post-registration qualification may enhance promotion prospects. For example, those wishing to become managers will undoubtedly benefit from a formal course in health-care management, although such a qualification may not be compulsory.

Others decide on post-registration training in order to 'round off' or add to their initial professional education. The motivation to expand education in this way is influenced by a number of specific and planned factors. For example, the person who intends to work in general management, research or education would profit from having a variety of training experiences of a relatively diverse nature. Conversely, one who intends to remain in clinical work either as a clinician or as a clinical manager, might decide to take one or two post-registration qualifications which relate to a specific area of clinical practice.

Continuing education

Continuing education, which includes post-registration study, encompasses all available professional educational experiences. It includes formal and informal experiences, the extent to which one has learned from day-to-day work, reading the professional literature, visits to centres of excellence, exchange of ideas with colleagues, and so on. Every work-place, irrespective of its quality, offers some opportunity for continuing education. Activities which may (or may not) be promoted by an employer include:

- Making library facilities available
- Organizing study days, conferences and discussion groups
- Seconding staff to courses
- Supporting staff to attend conferences, and to visit centres of excellence
- Encouraging and facilitating research
- Providing an environment conducive to the provision of high quality care
- Establishing links with relevant teaching and research institutions
- Attracting and retaining good staff.

The contribution of the employer inevitably requires the allocation of appropriate resources, something which may be difficult to achieve if funding is restricted (Dodwell, 1987). This contribution is, of course, a justified and necessary use of these resources which requires to be 'built on' by those who make use of them.

The ways in which the individual might contribute to education include:

- Reading the professional literature
- Contributing to the professional literature
- Attending and contributing to conferences etc.
- Visiting and learning from centres of excellence
- Making contact with colleagues who work elsewhere
- Understanding and making use of the research literature
- Contributing to the debate on professionalism and ethical issues.

Although the individual's contribution can be enhanced by a similar commitment from the organization, personal development is not totally dependant on the investment of resources by an employer. There is clearly much that can and should be done, even if little or no support is given. The ideal, and probably more usual, position is that a mutual participation by both the employer and employee exists in which each contributes resources of various kinds.

IDENTIFICATION OF CAREER PLANNING NEEDS

Having assessed previous development in terms of initial training, clinical experience, post-registration training, and continuing education it is now possible to identify present (immediate/short term) and future (medium-

and long-term) career needs. In order to identify priorities for the future, begin with a description of the strengths and weaknesses of current professional preparation. Discussing the subject with others who are more or less closely involved with your day-to-day work will be profitable (Chapter 20). The reason for including others in this evaluation is that it can be difficult to personally recognize, and occasionally difficult to admit to, professional strengths and weaknesses.

This summary, therefore, will contain a frank description of areas in which levels of knowledge or skill appropriate to present and future work have been achieved. For example, it might be concluded that keeping up-to-date with the professional literature by subscribing to a journal in a specialist area, and by reading the wider professional literature in the local library, is required. Conversely, you might feel that an area of weakness in clinical experience exists. For example, a present work position may require a firm understanding of hospice care provision; it is possible that this subject was not fully covered during training, and has not featured in subsequent clinical experience, or continuing/in-service education. An important deficit has therefore been identified. The outcome of this evaluation is written down, specific, includes a time frame, and is a realistic statement of personal professional strengths, and weaknesses. Because this evaluation will form the basis for much of future development, it is undertaken with both present and future in mind.

In identifying career planning needs and prioritizing them, ask the following questions:

Am I qualified to meet the demands of my present position, and what are my strengths and weaknesses in relation to it?

Prior to answering this, examine the present work position and make a list of the areas of skills and knowledge which are required. This is best done without any specific reference to existing personal skills and knowledge. As with other parts of this section, it is highly desirable that this question be answered in consultation with a colleague who can take an objective and informed view of the requirements of the job.

The next stage is to examine the 'check-list' of job requirements and to compare these with personal knowledge and skills levels. The participation of an informed colleague in this process will provide the opportunity for justifying a conclusion which indicates proficiency or deficiency in any particular item.

Is present career development activity contributing to meeting the demands of my present position?

This question is based on the realistic assumption that the answer to the first question concluded that there were one or more deficits in ability to meet the demands of a present job. It may well be that shortcomings have been previously recognized and that present career activity is 'making good' identified deficits. However, it is more likely that, following close scrutiny of existing skills and knowledge, areas have been identified which could be improved.

What are my future career plans?

Although career planning is a dynamic activity which is inevitably dependant on success being achieved during earlier stages, it is useful to visualize long-, medium- and short-term career possibilities. Although shorter term goals are easier to identify and achieve, make planning as long term as possible. Bearing in mind that short-term planning is the basis for medium-term planning, these should 'fit together' as much as possible. One way of looking at this topic is to begin with a distant point which may be some years away. If it is difficult to envisage a career goal which is so far in the future, then move back in time until a clear and identifiable career possibility is reached. For example, you might aspire to a life-long career in a senior clinical position, or identify a senior management position as being an appropriate goal in 10 or 15 years time.

To what extent do past and present experiences meet the requirements of future career plans?

Whereas the first question related to an ability to meet the demands of present employment, this question examines the extent to which past and present experiences give a preparation for future career development. Again, list the skills and knowledge which will be required to enable the meeting of the demands of future career plans, and examine these in terms of strengths and weaknesses.

PLANNING FOR MEETING IDENTIFIED NEEDS

Future plans take account of two principal factors; 'making good' deficits in previous training and experience, and planning to meet the needs of future changes in career direction. Both require the identification of means by which future training and experience can be used to meet these goals, confirming that personal and other resources are available, and placing in order to priority for the short, medium and long term.

Although some aspects of career development can, and should be, achieved in the long term, others are essential to a present position. The development of public speaking skills is a possible example of a medium-term goal for a recently qualified nurse; achieving an understanding of the principles of research might be seen as an urgent short-term goal for those who presently do not have this skill.

All plans must be specific and possible to achieve. Deciding to 'contribute to the professional literature and to seek opportunities to speak at conferences' is much more specific and appropriate than in deciding to 'make a greater contribution to the development of nursing'. Similarly, hoping to improve the general quality of the professional literature is something one cannot personally achieve, although you might contribute to the literature in your area of personal expertise.

Thus, goals for the future will be specific and possible to achieve within the constraints of personal and external resources. In personal terms, these constraints relate to individual abilities, and to resources such as time and finance. If it is decided to study for an academic qualification, ability and motivation are considered, as are the financial and time commitment of such an undertaking. In terms of external resources, constraints include the availability of the experience or training which has been identified, the ability of an employer to provide resources such as finances and/or time off work, and a range of practical issues which may prevent or enable reaching the identified goal.

IMPLEMENTATION OF CAREER PLANS

Having identified the plans, and made decisions about the way they will be reached, they are now implemented. Prior decisions concerning the urgency with which the goals should be reached will provide a time-frame for subsequent events. Adjustments to the plan will often have to be made for any of a number of reasons, including lack of external resources such as those required from an employer, and personal interests and opportunities.

EVALUATION OF CAREER PLANS

Evaluation is an ongoing activity which takes account of inevitable changing circumstances, personal needs and those of an employer, and which responds to impediments to reaching specific career goals. Some will be fully reached, others partially, some may have to be abandoned.

Some activities will be easier to evaluate than others, some will seem easy but will actually be more complex. If the need to read the professional literature has been identified, decisions have to be made about what this actually means. In order to evaluate the extent to which that goal has been met, decide if 'success' means subscribing to a journal, regular visits to the library, making use of literature at work, or all of these. A frank evaluation will prevent concluding that this goal has been reached as a result of reading one issue of one journal twice per year. Following assessment, identification, planning, implementation and evaluation the process returns to the starting point of further assessment.

CONCLUSION

The role of the professional nurse in career planning can be either an externalized or internalized one, depending on whether a reactive or proactive position is adopted. The externalized (reactive) position is one in which the individual reacts to external initiatives, pressures and expectations. Here, the person responds to opportunities (rather than makes them), and tends to look to others for career planning and development guidance. Success is viewed as largely relating to 'luck' and to 'being in the right place at the right time'. Success is also regarded as being wholly in the gift of significant others, rather than being strongly influenced by personal initiatives. The internalized (proactive) view of career planning is one which is entirely in keeping with the notion of professionalism; it causes you to seek out and make use of resources for professional growth. Thus the professional nurse will, with appropriate guidance from significant others, take personal responsibility for ensuring that all appropriate opportunities are taken.

The most obvious advantage of appropriate career planning is the increased quality of service provided. Throughout this text, another major advantage is also highlighted; the extent to which a successful career meets the needs of the individual. Such success has the potential to go some way toward satisfying all of the basic needs which were described by Maslow (1970) in his discussion of Motivation and Personality. Although a career is only a part of human experience, it can contribute much to satisfaction with life generally, and to the employee role in particular. The reverse position is true in that if a career does not contribute positively to meeting basis human needs, the outcome for the employee, the employer and for the consumer of the employee's services can at best be unsatisfying and, at worst, result in a poor quality of service. The remainder of this chapter, based on the work of Maslow (1970), summarizes the needs of the employee and how these might be met as a result of a successful career.

Physiological needs

'. . . are usually taken as the starting point for motivation. . .' (p. 35). They include the need for warmth, shelter, food and other items which give physiological sustinance.

In career terms, physiological needs are indirectly satisfied by income and other financial rewards derived from paid employment.

Safety needs

'. . . security; stability; dependency; protection; freedom from fear, from anxiety and chaos; need for structure, order, law, limits; strength in the protector; and so on' (p. 39).

These can be satisfied by the organizational structure within which you work, and by the extent to which use is made of the structure. Employer-related examples include providing security of employment, appropriate retirement benefits/arrangements, adequate orientation programmes, suitable staffing levels, clear operational policies, availability of an occupational health scheme, a safe working environment, and providing free access to relevant information. Employee-related examples include participating in continuing education opportunities, updating skills and knowledge, contributing to in-service education, raising issues for discussion, and drawing attention to environmental hazards.

Belongingness and love needs

Causing the person to seek '. . .affectionate relationships with people in general, namely, for a place in his group. . .' (p. 43).

These can be met by seeking to be, and being made to feel, part of a work group, having good working relationships with colleagues, and in working in an organization which encourages good peer group support, and satisfying employee/employer relationships.

Esteem needs

Esteem needs are reflected by individuals having '. . . the desire for strength, for achievement, for adequacy, for mastery and competence, for confidence in the face of the world, and for independence and freedom. Second, we have what we may call the desire for reputation or prestige (defining it as respect or esteem from other people), status, fame and glory, dominance, recognition, attention, importance, dignity or appreciation.' (p. 45).

Although an employer can contribute to meeting these needs, the individual plays a major part in terms of planning a career which will enable these to be met. Thus, the employee who fully participates in a range of professional activities will increase confidence and ability, the recognition of which by others (and the resultant 'feed-back') will satisfy self-esteem needs. Examples of these activities include achieving proficiency in clinical, research, management and teaching skills, reading and contributing to the professional literature, using continuing education opportunities, understanding and making use of research, and sharing knowledge with colleagues.

Self-actualization needs

These result from the person '. . .doing what he, individually, is fitted for. . .What a man can be, he must be.' (p. 46). An employer assists an employee to meet these needs by encouraging her (and making it possible) to make an optimal contribution to the work of the organization, by providing resources for full career development, and by encouraging the exercise of professional freedom and judgement. The employee contributes to meeting these needs by making full use of all career development opportunities which will enable her to function at the highest possible level.

In this chapter, a structure for planning a nursing career has been presented, a dynamic process in which all parts inter-relate. Because this type of planning is an integral part of professional development, and is of relevance throughout a career, I hope it will be used in one of two ways. First, by those who are entering nursing and need to consider how to plan a career. Second, by those who are already established in the profession and who may not have developed a structured and systematic career plan. In both instances, it is intended that this structure will be used as a starting point from which to continuously develop a career.

REFERENCES

Dodwell, M. (1987) An innovative training programme for ward sisters. *Journal of Advanced Nursing*, **12**, 311–19.
Ioannides, A. (1988) Assessing development. *Senior Nurse*, **8**(4), 31–3.
Jarczewski, P. (1986) The career plan. A luxury item? *Nursing Success Today*, **3**(10), 6–10.
Lathlean, J. (1986) Shock to the system. *Nursing Times*, **82**(49), 16–7.
Maslow, A. (1970) *Motivation and Personality*, 2nd edn, Harper and Row, New York.

Part Two

Chapter 8

Continuing education

DESMOND CORMACK

During initial training, students receive an education which enables them to function as professional nurses from the time of qualifying, and for a subsequent indefinite period without necessarily undertaking additional professional education. For some individuals, this may be as long as forty years; a position which may partly change if mandatory updating is introduced more widely. In practice, the content of initial training quickly becomes outdated as health science and nursing science knowledge increases. Additionally, many nurses follow a career path for which initial training is inadequate. Similarly, Christman (1987) suggested that: 'So rapid is the creation of new knowledge that many patients probably are being treated by obsolete methods every day.'

This situation is to be contrasted with that existing prior to the early 1960s when the speed of progress, and therefore the rather slow development of knowledge and skills, resulted in these being current for a relatively long period. In recognition of the rapid obsolescence of initial education individual nurses, the profession, and its registering bodies, have become more aware of the need for professional nurses to be commited to continuing education throughout a career.

Articles by Snell (1987) and Jarvis (1987) make specific reference to the notion of life-long professional education. In the United Kingdom and elsewhere this concept is embodied in the codes of professional conduct which registering bodies have constructed for application to all registered nurses, midwives and health visitors. For example, the United Kingdom Central Council For Nurses, Midwives and Health Visitors (UKCC) require these groups to 'Take every reasonable opportunity to maintain and improve professional knowledge and competence' (UKCC, 1984). Such a requirement, although not specifically defined, places a compulsory obligation on the individual for maintaining professional knowledge and competence levels. However, this chapter will address the issue from a rather wider perspective — that of professionalism. It will be assumed that, as implied by Jarvis (1987) 'life-long learning...is frequently regarded as an essential component of professionalism.' Indeed, it might be argued that a mandatory continuing education for nurses is redundant in that, by virtue of entering the profession, personal responsibility for maintaining professional knowledge and competence is automatically assumed. Kershaw (1985) reported that almost one-third of American states had legislation requiring nurses to produce evidence of having completed appropriate forms of continuing education as they re-licence for practice. Dodwell (1983) observed that although 19 states operated a mandatory continuing education policy, in many other states the policy was under review because of its value being uncertain. Kershaw (1985) also reported that it was still subject to considerable debate in terms of whether or not it should continue to be compulsory. Following a lecture tour of that country, Copperman (1987) expressed concern about the value of compulsory continuing education for nurses in the USA.

For some time, midwives in the UK have had a compulsory obligation to undertake periodic refreshment educational periods. In 1987 the United Kingdom Central Council For Nursing, Midwifery and Health Visiting published a discussion paper relating to mandatory periodic refreshment for nurses and health visitors (UKCC, 1987). The purpose of that paper was to enable informal discussion with the profession prior to drawing up actual proposals relating to mandatory continuing refreshment. The specific discussion points raised by the UKCC were:

1. Nurses and Health Visitors should undergo mandatory refreshment periods in order to maintain their professional competence.
2. Refreshment activities would include a mix of professional knowledge and aspects of general and specific areas of practice. These would have a number of specific outcomes relating to causing the individual to assess her educational needs and take personal responsibility for continuing education; promote professional growth and development; advance theoretical and practical knowledge in areas of practice; extend an understanding of research; increase knowledge of recent legislation which may affect practice.
3. Refreshment activities may be linked to a specific part of the Council's register and enable the person to maintain competence in that area of practice.
4. Evidence of successful completion of refreshment activities should be provided with each periodic payment of fees for registration. Employing authorities should provide a minimum of one day per year for refreshment activities in addition to existing orientation and inservice programmes.
5. The question of who should finance mandatory continuing education in terms of contributions by nurses and health visitors and/or their employer would need to be addressed.

Thus, the UKCC has expressed a firm commitment to the need for continuing education for nurses, a commitment which has professional relevance whether or not such education becomes mandatory.

SCOPE OF CONTINUING EDUCATION

Continuing education includes all educational experiences which enhance the knowledge and skills base of the individual. It ranges from the informal visit to a centre of excellence, to the formal type of study which is required to obtain a degree, additional registration or some other post-registration qualification for example. It also includes all professional experiences which are outwith 'normal' work activities. It includes attending an 'in-house' educational case conference, attending local study days, participating in national and international conference, and participating in local and national debates. It also includes more 'private' activities such as reading and writing for the professional literature, and evaluating and implementing current research. Although some of these activities are relatively difficult to quantify and, therefore, may not easily fit into a mandatory continuing education system, they are nevertheless important.

I will take a wide view of the concept of 'continuing education' and include virtually all of the material contained in this text. This broad approach places the subject more firmly within the context of a self-motivated process related to professionalism, and less closely allied to a mandatory activity which is subject to monitoring by registering bodies.

CONTINUING EDUCATION MOTIVATION

The underlying motivating principle in relation to continuing education is that knowledge and skills levels quickly become outdated, and that these can be maximized by a commitment to life-long updating within the context of continuing education, a principle which is fundamental to the concept of professionalism. One special feature of continuing professional education is that it takes place during adulthood. Benedict *et al.* (1984) presented a number of criteria which maximize the motivation of adults to learn. These criteria (which apply to adults generally) are of relevance to continuing education for nurses. Benedict *et al.* suggest that adults learn most effectively when: 'They feel the need to learn; an emotional and physical environment stimulates and supports the learning; they set personal goals for learning; they have been involved in the planning and operating of the learning experience; they are active participants in the learning process; their personal experience underpins the education; and responsibility for personal progress is shared with the teacher.'

Implicit in the views of Benedict *et al.* is the concept of internalized motivation to learn, such motivation to participate in continuing education being strongly linked to the concept of professionalism. Thus, the individual has a personal commitment to, and takes responsibility for, continuing education. This is to be contrasted with external motivation in which the individual participates in the process in order to satisfy the mandatory requirements of an employer or registering body. Internalized motivation will undoubtedly result in a more appropriate quality and quantity of continuing education which will go considerably beyond the minimum amount which is required by employers or other bodies.

There is evidence to suggest that nurses who become involved in continuing education activity prior to, or shortly after, initial training will develop a life-long commitment to it. In a review of the literature concerning the motivating factors which cause nurses to continue to learn, Millonig (1985) concluded that: 'The more education an individual has, the more frequently he or she participates in continuous learning activities.'

Thus, continuing education is a multi-purpose activity which relates to a number of facets of career development. Additionally, it can only realize its full potential if it is internally motivated and extends throughout the lifetime of a professional career.

CONTINUING EDUCATION PLANNING

As with career development generally, continuing education requires a structured and systematic plan. It is a continuous process in which you will review present status in relation to educational strengths and weaknesses, and identify short-, medium- and long-term goals. Although such a structure should be sufficiently flexible to accommodate changes in needs and opportunities, the following approach may be useful:

- Review present educational status with particular emphasis on previous professional education, relating this to current knowledge and skills.
- Identify educational gaps in relation to present (and future) areas of functioning.
- Analyse existing weaknesses, and identify educational opportunities which might be used to rectify these.
- Prioritize educational needs.
- Identify specific educational experiences and set personal goals in relation to these.
- Participate in these learning experiences.
- Evaluate the outcome of the learning experiences.
- Evaluate the learning experience in terms of the extent to which it has reduced the educational deficit.
- Review personal career development profile and identify future educational needs.

This approach to continuing education is a continuous one in which personal and professional needs are never fully satisfied. The prospect of becoming a 'perpetual student' may seen a daunting one, and making undue demands on personal time and energy. Indeed, it might be argued that the pressures which are generated by such an involvement may cause undue stress and 'burn-out' in a relatively short space of time. My own view coincides with that of Crotty (1987) who concluded that: 'Many studies suggest the positive effects of educational programmes to combat the burn-out syndrome.... It would appear that nurse education has a great part to play in the prevention of burn-out as all the potential causes discussed could be alleviated by the educational process'.

RESOURCES FOR CONTINUING EDUCATION

One resource required for successful continuing education is a personal commitment which is strongly influenced by the concept of professionalism; there are a number of others which require attention. The investment of personal time and energy is an important prerequisite. Additionally, a nurse may well invest a substantial amount of personal finance in the course of a career. There are, however, a number of external resources which might be reasonably expected, for example you should reasonably expect employers to be supportive (both in terms of time and finance). On occasions it might be appropriate for this support to be partial in that you and the employer share the cost. Even on these occasions when the employer apparently carries the 'full' cost in terms of time, you will invariably have to contribute some personal time to the endeavour.

Support may also be available from external agencies such as professional organizations, statutory bodies, charitable organizations and other groups. It is not unusual for outside bodies, including commercial organizations, to provide the cost of attendance at study days, conferences and other continuing educational activities. Requests for support can usually be maximized if you can convince the funding body that the experience will increase your contribution to the organization in which you work.

OPPORTUNITIES FOR CONTINUING EDUCATION

A range of continuing educational opportunities exist in relation to all personal and work environments, and in association with these. The key to success is in making use of these opportunities which can be either of the informal or formal type.

Informal continuing education

These opportunities, which may be self-generated or externally organized, include any educational activity which does not terminate in the award of a formal academic or professional qualification. The self-generated group includes reading, writing, professional visits or participation in informal discussions with colleagues. It also includes the setting up of journal clubs, discussion groups or any other educational forum where a group of nurses with similar educational needs meet to teach and learn from each other. Externally organized activities include participating in/contributing to study days, conferences which are offered by external bodies. Some short courses are of the informal type, a one-week introduction to research methods for example.

Staff/employer partnerships

Some employers provide an active in-service training programme, others require to be prompted by a clear expression of need by the nursing staff group. Such an approach will, in addition to making such a programme available, ensure that the content meets the specific needs of the participants. It is probable that a number of in-service activities have failed because of lack of attendance and interest resulting from inappropriate content. Duberley (1985) expresses it thus: '. . . the training and educational opportunities have been to a large extent determined by the needs of the employer. But there are gradual changes in this pattern. More and more one sees evidence of how the demands of the user — the qualified nurse — can shape the opportunities available.'

Clearly, there is scope for a partnership in which the needs of the employee and employer coincide in relation to continuing education. Skeath, Thorpe and Russell (1987) describe how a collaborative effort involving teaching and clinical staff constructed a successful continuing education project designed to meet specific needs relating to lifting patients, and to implementing the nursing process. Hoover (1987) described the development of a 'journal club' format in which nursing staff presented a journal article, nursing care plan, or topic of professional interest to colleagues. Clinical conferences which are a regular feature of postgraduate medical education are being increasingly used as an educational tool by nurses. Vousden (1985) outlined the means by which a group of charge nurses were involved in a programme designed to prepare them for participating in a changing philosophy of psychiatric nursing care. Stones (1986) used a research-based approach to determine the continuing education needs of nurses working in an intensive care unit.

Formal continuing education

In recent years many full-time and part-time educational opportunities for nurses have become available in both academic and professional subjects and in combinations of these. Generally, these are of the type which conclude with the award of a certificate, diploma, degree or some other formal confirmation of successful completion of a course of study. They might range in length from a three-month course on nursing administration, to a four-year part-time or full-time degree.

In relation to undertaking further clinically oriented post-registration education, consider the value of these to present and future career activity. For example, should a trained psychiatric nurse consider undertaking a further training in district nursing, health visiting or general nursing for example? Although there is a strong (and obvious) reason for taking further courses which will add to skills and knowledge base in the same specialty, the reasons for undertaking further courses of a very different nature are less obvious but, nevertheless, need to be considered. Additional courses in the same discipline, or a specialist aspect of it, are highly desirable and are generally encouraged (Brooking, 1985). Undertaking further courses in a different discipline can be of value to some individuals for a number of reasons. First, it might be desirable that those who aspire to a broad-based nurse management or advisory role have a good grounding in more than one major nursing discipline. For example, a senior nurse manager would benefit from having experience in hospital-based and community nursing. Second, you might make a conscious decision to equip yourself to work in more than one discipline in the course of a career in order to extend professional opportunities. Access to nursing and non-nursing academic courses of varying duration is reasonably open for most (if not all) nurses. The range of courses extends from those subjects which are normally taken at school (English, mathematics, biology, chemistry for example) to degree and higher degree opportunities. Availability is greatest in the major conurbations, although distance learning, local evening classes and a general increase in local educational opportunities have increased access in recent years. The justification for undertaking continuing education of an academic (or academic/professional) nature are well documented. Important aspects of that argument include increased academic credibility, making the profession more attractive to educationally able entrants, equality with other professions such as medicine, increased knowledge and clinical, research, educational and management competence, the development of an autonomous nursing role, increased professional prestige, and increased assertiveness and 'political' skill (Brooking, 1985 and *Nursing Standard*, 1988). It is not this author's aim to claim that all the present 'ailments' associated with the nursing profession will be remedied by a general increase in the academic abilities of its members. Rather, it is suggested that such an ability is more frequently accepted as the 'norm' and that it has much to contribute to individual and collective development of professionalism.

WHO PAYS FOR CONTINUING EDUCATION?

There are two major costs involved in all continuing education activities: time and money. At the one extreme, you may have to pay with personal time and money. At the other extreme, an employer or alternative

funding agency may provide both. Very often, a mixture of self/employer/
external agency support is available. Some employers have a substantial
continuing education budget, others have little or nothing. Tyler (1987)
suggested that the UKCC, or the professional body of which she was a
member, should meet the costs. Horne (1987) who conducted a small-scale
survey of opinion relating to who should pay continuing education costs,
reported that individuals felt they should share the responsibility for their
own continuing education and that, in addition to salary, they should
receive a continuing education grant. Additionally, it was suggested that
employers should allocate specific time to be allocated for this purpose
(Horne, 1988).

Many centres of higher education insist that academic staff participate
fully in continuing education, one of the reasons being that the institution
may lose its 'licence to teach' if its staff group are not regularly updated.
The employers in such centres, therefore, have an obvious vested interest
in providing reasonable support and funding for staff, and in providing
access to a range of continuing education opportunities. At present, no
such requirement formally exists in many of the areas/institutions in which
professional nurses work. However, it may be that employers of nurses
should be subjected to the same requirement and that the 'institution'
shares the responsibility with the individual nurse.

Given the essential nature of continuing education, and the benefits
which accrue to the individual and employer, it might be reasonable to
expect that both will share the cost. Because of their recognition of the
importance of continuing education, employers are becoming more able
and willing to provide appropriate levels of support.

Clearly, there is considerable conflict in views relating to 'who pays for
continuing education', a debate which has become much more focused
since the UKCC published its discussion paper on mandatory periodic
refreshment (UKCC, 1987). It may be that an employer, or some other
agency, might be expected to pay for the suggested mandatory minimum
of one-day refreshment per year. However, this could raise, rather than
solve, at least two problems. First, some employers might adhere to funding the mandatory minimum of, for example, one day per year. Second,
some nurses might only opt to be involved in continuing education for that
relatively limited period.

One view is that, in large part, continuing education should remain a
collaborative effort involving the individual and employer, and that it
should not be constrained within relatively narrow mandatory limits.
Convincing arguments for support can be made by individuals, collective
arguments and pressures can and should come from employee groups,
professional organizations and trade unions, and from bodies such as the
UKCC. In relation to such a employee/employer partnership, this author

agrees with Barnes (1985) who observed that continuing education costs money and, like all services, management have to see some sort of return for its investment.

LEARNING ABOUT CONTINUING EDUCATION OPPORTUNITIES

Self-generated opportunities such as meeting with an 'expert' or visiting a centre of excellence normally come to attention by word of mouth, or by reading a report of an area or activity of interest. Having a good professional network, and regularly reading the nursing press enables the identification of such areas or individuals. In relation to setting up a local activity such as a journal club, seminar or workshop, close contact and exchange with colleagues in your discipline will help identify educational needs which can be met on a group basis (Chapter 20).

Activities organized by other agencies can only be identified by a combination of reading and personal enquiry. In-service programmes are probably the easiest to find out about; read the notice boards, read internal memos and newsletters, and talk to in-service education staff. The local press often carries notice of such things and open lectures, presentations for people with a special interest in such subjects as the community care of the elderly, and meetings of local groups of health care staff. Professional organizations such as the Royal College of Nursing organize local, regional, national and international events which are usually advertised in the nursing press, in addition to being made known to individual members. The nursing press generally is probably the best source of information on a variety of continuing education opportunities, as are the specialist journals of other health care related disciplines such as social work, clinical psychology, physiotherapy, occupational therapy and medicine.

The UKCC and the four National Boards approve a wide range of courses and provide details of the course types, duration, and addresses from which further information can be obtained. Details of academic or academic/professional courses can be obtained from the many universities, polytechnics and central institutions which offer these. Access to such information can normally be obtained in either a college of nursing library, or in the higher education sector libraries. Local education authorities will be able to provide full details of academic courses.

CONTRIBUTING TO CONTINUING EDUCATION OF OTHERS

All forms of continuing education depend heavily on contributions from a range of 'teachers', many of whom teach on an informal basis. The success of such programmes requires that every nurse (all of whom have something to teach others) be willing to contribute. This sharing of knowledge and skill is a central part of professionalism. Many preregistration programmes cultivate this teaching ability in learners by expecting them to present discussion topics, participate in a professional article presentation, and lead case presentations. Indeed, an important part of the qualified nurse's role is to teach patients, learners and other unqualified staff. It is a natural expectation, therefore, that these skills be further used to teach others. Thus, many forms of continuing education require that today's student is tomorrow's teacher (Chapter 12).

THE BEGINNING AND END OF CONTINUING EDUCATION

One widely held view of continuing education, in terms of when it begins and ends, is that it '. . . is a life-long learning process which builds on and modifies previously acquired knowledge, skills and attitudes of the individual' it '. . . consists of planned learning experiences beyond a basic nursing educational program' (American Nurses' Association, 1974).

However, although it must take place after pre-registration education, there are strong reasons for suggesting that it should start at the beginning of that education, and that it be a normal expectation of students on entry to that education. Clarke (1985) proposed that a commitment to career-long learning be instilled from the outset, in schools of nursing, an approach which has much to commend it from several viewpoints. First, teaching staff are ideally placed to encourage and expect learners to participate in educational opportunities beyond those which are a 'compulsory' part of initial nurse training. By so doing, they will assist learners to develop a life-long commitment to continuing education. Indeed, it might be unreasonable to expect learners to suddenly take a personal responsibility in this respect after a number of years in which others (teachers) take much of the responsibility and initiative. Fortunately, the reality is that initial training provides a basis from which the emergent professional nurse takes on a commitment to life-long continuing education.

Just as the starting point for continuing education is evident, on entry to an initial training programme, the end point is equally clear; the end of a professional nursing career. Such a life-long participation is necessary to ensure that the individual is fully equipped in terms of knowledge, skill and competence.

REFERENCES

American Nurses' Association (1974) Standards for continuing education in nursing. *Journal of Continuing Education in Nursing*, **5**(3), 32–9.
Barnes, S. (1985) Never too old to learn. *Nursing Mirror*, **161**(4), 48–9.
Benedict, D., Collier, F., Masar, B. and Wilkinson, L. (1984) *Learning a Living in Canada* (Vol. 1) Report to the Minister of Employment and Immigration, Canada.

Brooking, J. (1985) Advanced psychiatric nursing education in Britain. *Journal of Advanced Nursing*, **10**, 455–68.

Christman, L. (1987) The future of the nursing profession. *Nursing Administration Quarterly*, **11**(2), 1–8.

Clarke, M. (1985) The use of research reports in planning continuing education for trained nurses. *Journal of Advanced Nursing*, **10**, 475–82.

Copperman, H. (1987) Continuing education: An American experience (letter). *Nursing Times*, **83**(38), 14.

Crotty, M. (1987) 'Burnout' and its implications for the continuing education of nurses. *Nurse Education Today*, **7**, 278–84.

Dodwell, M. (1983) In service training (1), continuing education in the USA *Nursing Times*, **79**(24), 24–6.

Duberley, J. (1985) Continuing education — Whose responsibility? *The Professional Nurse*, **1**(1), 4–6.

Hoover, J. (1987) Promoting self-directed enquiry. *The Professional Nurse*, **2**(11), 361–62.

Horne, E.M. (1987) Mandatory continuing education: Your chance to respond. *The Professional Nurse*, **3**(2), 55–7.

Horne, E.M. (1988) Mandatory continuing education: Your views. *The Professional Nurse*, **3**(5), 162–4.

Jarvis, P. (1987) Lifelong education and its relevance to nursing. *Nurse Education Today*, **7**(2), 49–55.

Kershaw, B. (1985) A lesson from America. *Nursing Times*, **81**(6), 41–7.

Millonig, V. (1985) Motivational orientation toward learning after graduation. *Nursing Administration Quarterly*, **9**(4), 79–86.

Nursing Standard (1988) Who me — a degree? *Nursing Standard*, **2**(20), 24–5.

Skeath, B., Thorpe, E. and Russell, L. (1987) Alternative approaches. *Senior Nurse*, **7**(4), 43–4.

Snell, J. (1987) Enter the life-long learner? *Nursing Times*, **83**(38) 19.

Stones, J.N. (1986) A survey of continuing educational needs of nurses working in an intensive care unit. *Intensive Care Nursing*, **1**(3), 130–37.

Tyler, P. (1987) Refresher courses (letter). *Nursing Times*, **83**(45), 15.

United Kingdom Central Council for Nursing, Midwifery and Health Visiting (1984) *Code of Professional Conduct*. United Kingdom Central Council for Nursing, Midwifery and Health Visiting, London.

United Kingdom Central Council for Nursing, Midwifery and Health Visiting (1987) *Mandatory Periodic Refreshment for Nurses and Health Visitors (Discussion Paper)*. United Kingdom Central Council for Nursing, Midwifery and Health Visiting, London.

Vousden, M. (1985) Taking the strain. *Nursing Mirror*, **161**(7), 25–8.

Chapter 9

Nursing research

DESMOND CORMACK

Research is thus not a luxury for the academic, but a tool for developing the quality of nursing decisions, prescriptions and actions. Whether as clinicians, educators, managers or researchers we have a research responsibility; neglect of that responsibility could be classified as professional negligence.

(McFarlane of Llandaff, 1984, p. xi)

Research may be defined as a planned and systematic collection and analysis of information (data) for the purpose of seeking answers to specific questions and thereby increasing nursing knowledge. It is a crucial part of the continuing education and career development of *all* nurses. During the past twenty years, when research has been widely discussed both nationally and internationally, the question has often been asked: 'What can nursing research do and what is its significance to nursing practice, management and education?' The generally accepted answer to that question is that nursing research can:

- optimize the quantity and quality of nursing care, management and education;
- establish scientifically based principles for nursing practice, management and education;
- initiate and develop constructive critical thinking in nurse clinicians, managers and teachers;
- enable identification of the positive aspects of nursing activity which need further development;
- enable identification and modification of those areas of nursing practice, management and education which are ineffective;
- enable optimal use to be made of limited resources;
- provide evidence which will support resource demand;
- enable the construction of a professional and academic basis for nursing as a profession by the creation of scientifically based knowledge and skills.

The purpose of nursing research, therefore, is to enable all activity to be based on sound scientific principles rather than on tradition, convention and personal opinions. Because nursing has only recently started to develop in terms of research, there are many questions which are still unanswered from a research viewpoint. Indeed, many of the questions relevant to nursing have not yet been identified and asked. Nursing research seeks to answer those questions which are relevant to activities for which nurses have a major responsibility, or which relate to the staff group (nurses) who undertake these activities. For example, it might be concerned with the way in which we prevent pressure sores, reduce patient's anxiety, assess nursing care needs, control pain by means of nursing intervention, achieving an understanding of the means by which we communicate with our patients, or methods by which we can understand and control aggressive behaviour. Areas of research relevant to nurse education include an examination of the relationship between nursing theory and practice, comparisons of differing educational methods, and studies of how best to teach a particular subject area such as the use of the nursing process. Areas relevant to nursing administration include an examination of the use of manpower planning strategies, a study of sickness/absence levels in a given staff group, or the study of environmental design as it relates to patient care and nursing activity.

Although many nurses subscribe to the view that nursing should become a research based profession, there is often some confusion as to how this general aim relates to individuals. Clearly, not all nurses will become researchers and develop the skills necessary to understand *and* do research. However, there are other levels of knowledge and understanding which are required by every nurse in order to understand and (where appropriate) make use of the research. Although some readers may wish to develop the knowledge and skills required to do research, this chapter is primarily directed at clinicians, managers and teachers who wish to develop a sufficient understanding of the principles of research to enable them to understand and make use of it in the course of their work. In order for nursing to become a research based profession, it is necessary that all nurses must be able to:

1. read, interpret and apply research in their own specialist area, keep up to date with contemporary research, and make use of research findings in order to make decisions about professional practice;
2. identify and discuss areas in which research can contribute to professional practice. Practitioners, be they clinicians, educators or managers are in the best position to identify those areas in which research requires to be conducted;
3. help patients who are subjects of research to understand the implications and consequences of that involvement. Just as patients look to nurses to help them understand the nature of their illness and treatment, they will wish to discuss their involvement in research with nurses;

4. give free and informed assistance to researchers, and give as much assistance as is possible, particularly where there is patient involvement; and
5. understand and apply ethical concepts relating to nursing research, particularly where those relate to research which involves patients.

Nurse managers must be able to:

1. monitor nursing research which has been conducted in their area of responsibility, ensuring that it is being properly conducted and that nursing and other resources which are being used are not detracting from the quality of patient care;
2. identify those areas in which nursing research is required and give appropriate support to those who are undertaking it;
3. create an environment in which 'research mindedness' is encouraged. Where necessary, this will involve the allocation of resources to those who are undertaking research; and
4. be aware of all resources (including human, financial and technological) which are assistive to research activity.

Nurse teachers must be able to:

1. identify and make use of research which is relevant to nurse education;
2. expose students to the research which is relevant to the subject being taught;
3. teach students how to incorporate research findings into their examinations, coursework and clinical practice;
4. generate research mindedness in students; and
5. be sufficiently aware of the research process to teach students how to understand and make use of it.

THE RESEARCH PROCESS

Although the potential exists for all professional nurses to carry out small-scale research projects in the course of their career, it is recognized that, because of the early stage of development of nursing as a research based profession, only a minority of nurses will become researchers. For readers who wish to become sufficiently aware of the research process to enable them to undertake a research based study under supervision, they are referred to Cormack (1984). A general understanding of the research process is essential for all nurses in order to enable individual pieces of research to be understood and (where appropriate) implemented. It is intended that the following overview of the subject (Figure 9.1) will pro-

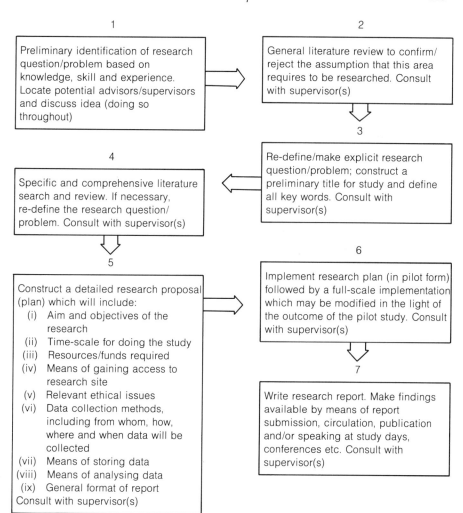

Figure 9.1 The research process (an overview).

vide a basis from which to *begin* to understand what research is, and to enable evaluation of individual studies.

1. Preliminary identification of research question/problem

All research begins with observation and consideration of previous professional experience, knowledge and skill. These may relate to personal functioning or that of other individuals, groups or systems. The research question/problem is usually identified as a result of a 'hunch' that a particular area of practice, management or education requires to be closely examined from a research viewpoint. Although research is firmly based on the scientific method, without these intuitive feelings or hunches specific areas of research would not commence. These intuitive feelings develop as a result of having a questioning attitude towards all areas of professional functioning. At this point the researcher has no more than a general hunch that a particular area requires to be researched. It is essential that these views are fully discussed with colleagues who have a knowledge of the subject area, and with potential research supervisors. The question of research supervision is a fundamental one which permiates throughout the entire research process.

Next, write down in clear and precise terms exactly which questions are to be asked, and/or which problem(s) are to be solved. Clarifying the purpose of a research study is one of the most difficult steps in the process, but which requires to be well done as early as possible.

2. General literature review

It may well be that the questions/problems identified in the initial phase of the research process have already been thoroughly researched. One way of determining whether or not this is so is to undertake a general (although thorough) review of the existing research literature. Such a review will enable confirmation or rejection of the initial assumptions which indicated that this particular area requires to be researched.

3. Re-define/make explicit research question/problem

Assuming that the general literature review indicates that the subject has not been researched previously, or has not been examined from this particular point of view, the research question/problem is made more explicit and each of its elements fully defined. Create a preliminary title for the study and define all key words in it. For example, the title 'A study of hand-washing techniques used by surgical ward nurse' will be further defined by giving a detailed explantation of the words 'hand-washing', 'techniques', 'surgical', 'ward' and 'nurses'. The general aims and specific objectives of the study are then identified, and are accompanied by a detailed description of the nature of the identified question/problem, and a convincing argument as to why this particular subject requires to be researched.

4. Specific and comprehensive literature search and review

A specific search and review of the relevant literature is undertaken next. The literature is looked at from the point of view of the specific subject to be studied, as is the appropriate scientific background, and the methods used in previous work. This review is important for three reasons. First, it ensures that you have a comprehensive knowledge of the subject to be investigated, or at least appreciate the extent of the knowledge which is required for such research. Second, it may be discovered that a very similar study to the one you are planning has already provided a complete or partial answer to the question which is being asked in this study. In which case you might decide to abandon this particular avenue of research, or to modify it. Third, it may be decided to replicate a previous study, rather than carry out an original piece of research. Such replication is perfectly reasonable and enables comparisons and confirmation to be made.

Defining the research area and reviewing the literature are closely related. The literature search is focused on the area which is thought to be a problem, it also generates research questions and/or substantially modifies these. At this stage three important questions are answered before proceeding; these are: *What would be the value of this study? Does it need to be done?* and *Do I have sufficient motivation to research this particular area?*

5. Construct a detailed research proposal

The construction of a detailed research proposal (plan) will provide a blueprint for undertaking the research study. In addition to acting as a guide for the research, the proposal has a number of other functions such as being a requirement for obtaining funding and other resources, it is discussed by research and ethics committees, and will be examined by those individuals and/or organizations from whom you request permission to gather data. See Pollock and Tilley (1988) for a discussion of the work of the ethics committee. The specific elements of a research proposal are:

i. Aim and objectives of the research

The general aim of the research is clearly stated and discussed in some detail. Readers of the proposal should be in no doubt as to what the research is intended to achieve, and must be convinced of the appropriateness and value of the study. The objectives of the study usually consist of a discussion of all specific sub-parts of the general aim. Thus, the aim is a broad statement of intent; the objectives are much more detailed and specific.

ii. Time-scale

A preliminary time-scale for undertaking the entire study is prepared in some detail. The timetable includes all parts of the research process from the undertaking of a comprehensive and specific literature review, to the writing up of the research report. Although flexible, the research timetable includes a realistic description of all time which is to be spent on the study. A typical time-scale for undertaking any piece of research will devote approximately one-quarter of the total time to each of the following parts; reviewing the literature, collecting data, analysing data, and writing up the final report. An important function of this timetable is to enable you to work within a specific time-frame and to ensure that the task is complete in a well prescribed time limit.

iii. Resources/funds required

The types of resources and funding required by a particular piece of research are varied and depend on a number of factors relating to how and where the data will be collected. In addition to personal time you may require funding for typing, postage, printing, travel, telephone calls, equipment, specialist statistical advice, specialist data collection tools and textbooks.

iv. Means of gaining access to research site

Permission to gather data is sought from a range of individuals and/or organizations. For example, you may have to obtain permission from an appropriate research and ethics committee, the administrative staff of the organization concerned, and from the individuals who are to be the subjects of the study. See Cormack (1980) and Wilson-Barnett (1984) for a fuller discussion of this subject.

v. Relevant ethical issues

Irrespective of the nature of the research, every researcher must seriously consider a range of ethical issues. Additionally, nurses working in areas in which research is being undertaken, and nurses in managerial positions also have such responsibilities. The Royal College of Nursing (1977) in its publication *Ethics Related to Research in Nursing* presented the following guidelines for nurses undertaking or associated with research.

> The researcher has obligations to the subjects of study, to sponsors/ employers, to colleagues and to the development and promotion of knowledge.... The nurse researcher must possess knowledge and skills compatible with the demands of the investigation to be undertaken and must recognise and not overstep the boundaries of his/her research competence. He/she should not accept work he/she is not qualified to carry out. (Those learning to do research should only work under the guidance of an experienced researcher.) Nurses in authority in places where research is to be undertaken have obligations to the subjects of the study, to the governing body of the institution or place of work, to the sponsors of the study and to the research worker. Nurses practicing in places where research is being carried out have obligations

to patients/clients and to the development and promotion of knowledge through research. When assisting in the conduct of research they have obligations to adhere to the ethical code binding upon all research workers.

vi. Data collection methods

This section of the proposal describes, in detail, the research methodology which is to be used. This area, which is potentially the most difficult of all aspects of the research process, requires that the methodology be based on firm scientific principles which will ensure that the results are both valid and reliable. The researcher decides on the most appropriate type of research, for example, descriptive or experimental, or a combination of the two. The data collection methods to be used will vary depending on the type and purpose of the research but may include observation, interviewing, the use of questionnaires, or one or more of the many other data collection techniques which are available. Decisions are made regarding the population or sample from whom data are to be collected, and as to how, where and when the data will be gathered.

vii. Means of storing data

Decisions regarding how the data will be stored for subsequent analysis are also made at this stage. Some data are stored in their original form and analysed manually; other types of data (particularly the large quantitative type) may be stored on a computer which will assist in subsequent complex analyses. If data are to be stored on a computing system, full discussion with an expert in that area takes place at this point. Legal aspects of data storage will require full consideration (Chapter 11).

viii. Means of analysing data

Well in advance of collecting the data decisions are made with regard to the type of analyses which will be made. Depending on the type of analysis which is thought to be required, it may or may not be necessary to consult a statistician.

ix. General format of report

Early decisions with regard to the possible format of the report will guide the researcher in terms of data collection, decisions about analysis, and provide a structure for the subsequent writing up phase of the research process. Indeed, it is possible to begin to write up part of the first draft of the final research report very early on in the study. For example, it is quite usual to write those sections relating to the research question, background to the research, and the review of the literature even before data are collected.

6. Implement research proposal (plan)

Prior to implementing the full research plan, it is usual to undertake a small-scale pilot study which may, for example, be applied to 5 or 10% of the population or sample which will eventually be used. The purpose of the pilot study is to test out the research plan and to ensure that the correct type of data can be collected, analysed and contribute to an understanding of the question/problem being studied. If the pilot study identifies particular problems with the research method it is necessary to go 'back to the drawing board' and modify the project and re-submit it to a further pilot study. Following a successful pilot study, the full study is carried out.

7. Write research report

All pieces of research conclude with a written report which is then made available in a number of formats. This 'publication' of the research may take the form of a submission to a particular individual or organization, restricted or general circulation of the report, publication in the professional journals, or speaking at study days, conferences or with colleagues. The purpose of a research report is to make known the findings of the study and to inform others as to how it was carried out in order that they can assess the value of the work, use similar methods for their own research, and enable others to avoid the mistakes which are occasionally made.

RESEARCH REPORT STRUCTURE

Although there are obviously differences in the detailed structure and content of every research report, the following general structure is typical of many, and is one which you might generally expect to find.

- A detailed statement of the purpose of the study and of the question/ problem which is being addressed.
- A comprehensive critical analysis of the reviewed literature.
- The means of gaining access to the research site.
- Details of the research method used and the reasons for deciding against other possible methods.
- The sample size and response rate. That is, how many people or organizations took part in the study and how many were asked to do so.
- Discussion of the ethical issues involved in the study.
- A full description of the data storage and analysis methods.
- A description of the pilot study/studies and any major changes which resulted from these.
- Copies of all relevant documentation such as questionnaires, interview schedules, or observation recording sheets.

- A full presentation and discussion of the research findings, including the statistical data from which conclusions were made.
- A full discussion of the extent to which the study contributed to research based nursing knowledge as applied to clinical practice, management or education.
- The limitations of the study, and any mistakes which were identified with the benefit of hindsight.
- Questions raised by the research and specific recommendations for future research in this particular area.

EVALUATING PUBLISHED RESEARCH

A primary function of all pieces of research is to enable others to read it, evaluate it and (when applicable) implement it. In order to make a judgement with regard to the quality of an individual study, it is necessary to undertake a systematic evaluation of it. On occasions, you are restricted to a summary of the work, usually in the form of a journal article, rather than having access to the entire report. If the material is available in a reduced or summarized form, obtain and read the entire document before seriously considering its implementation. The following discussion of evaluation will be based on the assumption that the full report is available. However, it is recognized that you may frequently only have access to limited material, for example in the form of one or more journal articles.

The researcher

The credentials, background and experience of the researcher goes some way towards determining the credibility of the research. For example, a study undertaken by an inexperienced person as part of a learning process is of less value than one undertaken by a post-doctoral researcher working alone or in collaboration with other experienced workers. It is not being suggested that small research studies undertaken by inexperienced workers are of no value.

Research title

The title of the study should be a fair and accurate reflection of the intention of the researcher. Confusing or inappropriate titles may well reflect a similarly confusing approach to the study. You should reasonably expect that the title of the report will accurately and clearly reflect its content.

Aim and objectives

The early part of the report must contain a specific and clear description of the overall aim and specific objectives of the research. This section should leave you in absolutely no doubt with regard to the purpose of the study and should be fully supported by the convincing argument of the need for this particular study being undertaken. Some studies are descriptive in nature, describing events, activities or some other phenomena. Others are experimental in nature and involve manipulating and/or changing natural phenomena and comparing the outcome with near identical phenomena which have been unchanged. This section of the report should make an absolutely clear and concise statement with regard to the research approach which is to be used.

Literature review

This section must convince you that a comprehensive search of the literature has been undertaken and should present a critical evaluation of the published literature. You expect more than a statement or summary of the content of previously published literature; and also expect to have it critically analysed in term of its relevance, strengths and weaknesses. If recent literature on the subject matter exists, it should be included. Finally, the reviewed literature should be relevant to the aim and objectives of this particular study.

Ethical issues

The Royal College Of Nursing (1977) gives a detailed account of ethical issues which relate to nurses undertaking research. That report recommended that nurse researchers should:

1. Be satisfied that the knowledge sought is not already available. However, it is perfectly legitimate for researchers to replicate previous studies in order to determine their reliability, and for other purposes;
2. Ensure that free and informed consent is obtained from the subjects of the study. If the nature of the research is such that fully informing subjects before the study would invalidate the results, then whatever explanation is possible should be given;
3. Explain to subjects how their names came to the knowledge of the researcher;
4. Ensure that subjects are protected against physical, mental, emotional or social injury;
5. Adhere to promises of confidentiality and/or anonymity;
6. Be aware of the dangers of raising false hopes or unnecessary anxieties;
7. Where appropriate, receive the approval of the relevant ethics/research committees;
8. Have the necessary skills and knowledge to undertake the piece of research. Where necessary, researchers should work under the supervision of an experienced researcher;

9. Recognize personal limitations in terms of knowledge and skill;
10. Publish or otherwise make available the results of the research;
11. Recognize and report the limitations of the research;
12. Acknowledge the contribution of others who participated in the research, and the subjects of the study;
13. Make reasonable attempts to ensure that the research is read and used by others. Recognize a responsibility for the advancement of nursing theory and research method;
14. Adhere to a professional code of ethics as they relate to nursing research;
15. Avoid interference in professional patient/nurse relationships;
16. Where action research is used, interaction between the researcher and subjects must be mutually agreed.

Research plan

This section provides a detailed account of all further aspects of the research programme including the methods to be used, size of sample, and method of entry to the research site. The researcher should provide a convincing argument for the use of selected data collection techniques. These should, of course, be appropriate to the questions which are being addressed in the study. Readers will be concerned with the size of the sample and the extent to which the results can be generalized to a larger population. The means of selecting the sample is also of interest in terms of whether subjects were self-selected, or whether they were randomly selected.

Pilot study

It is normal to undertake a pilot study in order to ensure that the proposed plan is operable. Details of the outcome of such a pilot study, and subsequent adjustments to the plan, are reported in full.

Data collection

This section describes the implementation of the research plan and includes all detail relating to the means by which data were actually collected and associated problems (if any). Subjects' response rate is given.

Analysis of data

Two kinds of statistics are applied to the analysis of data: descriptive and comparative/inferential. Although a discussion of statistical analysis is outside the scope of this text brief comments will be made on these two types.

Descriptive statistics are those which describe data and draw conclusions from it. For example, if 100 subjects are asked a particular question, the results might be presented as 25% of respondents said 'Yes', 70% of respondents said 'No', and the remainder replied 'Don't know'. These statistics merely describe the data.

Inferential statistics, which are more difficult although not impossible to understand, apply specific statistical tests to the data in order to make inferences. Readers who have little or no statistical knowledge may be tempted to assume that the correct inferential statistical tests have been applied and the correct conclusions made. Such readers would be well advised to consult with a colleague who has knowledge of inferential statistics before assuming that they have been correctly used. See Reid and Boore (1987) for a comprehensive discussion of statistical analysis.

Another form of analysis, which is also beyond the scope of this text, is the qualitative approach which relies less on numerical forms of data, and which attempts to seek relationships between pieces of information and to draw appropriate conclusions. As with inferential statistical analysis, readers who are not familiar with this research approach and subsequent analysis of data should consult with someone who has appropriate expertise. See Akinsanya (1988) for a discussion of quantitative and qualitative research.

Conclusions

Conclusions are stated clearly and are related to the aim and objectives of the study. Ideally, each of the objectives of the research should have a corresponding conclusion in which the researcher describes the outcome. Just as the data should reflect each of the objectives of the study, each part of the study should have a corresponding conclusion. It is usual for researchers to present individual conclusions which relate to each of the objectives, and follow this with a general conclusion which relates to the overall aim of the study. Finally, the conclusions must be firmly based on, and supported by, the data which are presented in the study.

General points regarding evaluation

Are the researcher's personal views/opinions clearly separated from the actual findings of the research? Does the study have implications for nursing practice, management or education? When did the study take place? Does the study contribute to the advancement of nursing knowledge and/ or skill? Is the report readable and one which can be understood by the target readership?

The success of a piece of research depends on the quality of the work, the researcher's ability to communicate with potential consumers of the research, and the ability of nurses to read, understand and evaluate the study. Traditionally, nursing research has been surrounded (wrongly) by an aura of mystique which causes some non-research nurses to have difficulty in digesting many research reports. Fortunately, this position is now changing rapidly with nurses generally having a sufficient understanding of the research process to enable them to make a critical evaluation of research reports. However, it is still the case that some researchers produce reports which are incomprehensible to the average reader. If such a report is encountered, assume that the researcher, and possibly even the research, is suspect. Understanding the research process, which was outlined earlier in this chapter, is an essential prerequisite to making a critical evaluation of individual studies. The following section describes some of the means by which such an understanding can be achieved.

LEARNING ABOUT RESEARCH

As with other issues dealt with in this text, learning about research is part of a life-long and continuing process which begins during initial training and ends at the termination of a professional nursing career. As with other topics, it is not a 'one off' learning experience which takes place during a discrete period, for example by attending a one-week introduction to nursing research course.

Pre-registration training

Pre-registration training provides two bases for developing research mindedness. First, it provides the clinical base upon which all subsequent nursing research is founded. Second, it provides a range of exposures to the principles and use of nursing research. These include:

- the provision of well-stocked libraries (and a skilled librarian) which will enable students to gain access to all published materials with a research base. An important part of this provision is the availability of nursing indexes, bibliographies and other means of 'searching' the literature (see Chapter 10 for a full discussion of this subject);
- an education which is research based and in which teachers make reference to published research materials as they relate to nursing practice, management and education;
- initiating discussion of published research as it relates to the particular subject being taught. Students are now expected to incorporate research findings into their clinical and other discussion presentations;
- research papers being part of the reading material which is prescribed by teaching staff; and
- introduction to the research process and discussion of selected data collection methods.

All of the above items are now a normal and natural part of initial nurse training and represent an important means by which the nursing profession is becoming research based.

Research in the workplace

Many opportunities exist in the place of employment which will enable the continued development of research knowledge and (possibly) skill. These opportunities develop from, and are a continuation of, those which are available during initial training.

Resource persons who have a knowledge of the research process are usually available in places of employment. Ideally, there will be a nurse colleague with such knowledge; invariably there will be members of other staff groups such as medicine or psychology who have research skills. My experience has been that such resource persons, whether or not they are nurses, are willing to assist individual nurses to develop their knowledge and experience of research. In addition to contributing to an understanding of research generally, such persons might be used for giving specific advice on matters such as the statistical analysis of data in published research reports.

Many hospitals and community care organizations have some ongoing research projects from which individual nurses can learn, if not contribute to. Involvement in such a project is an important means of learning. Additionally, the existence of such research activity helps to promote a general feeling of research mindedness among the staff group.

Some health care organizations and places of employment are now producing a policy statement outlining their research strategy. Such a policy may relate to the health care professions generally, or to each of the disciplines including nursing. When moving to a new place of employment, it is reasonable to ask whether or not the organization has a clearly developed strategy relating to nursing research.

Research journal clubs/discussion groups enable participants to learn about research methods, and to develop an understanding of the research which relates to their particular specialty. These activities, which are often self-generated by the staff, may be multidisciplinary and involve medical staff, psychologists, social workers, nurses and others. In the absence of this activity, or if nurses have no access to it, it is usual for a nursing staff group to initiate it in the form of continuing education activity.

In-service education provision relating to the understanding and implementation of nursing research is an important resource for learning about the subject. In the absence of 'in-house' nursing staff with appropriate experience, these can be hired in or, alternatively, staff from other disciplines can be recruited.

Research and ethics committees now usually have a nurse member.

'Research' is now part of the vocabulary of all the health care professions. New developments are becoming research based in order to maximize the quantity and quality of clinical practice, management and education.

The employee/employer collaboration in developing research activity reflects the view of McFarlane (1984) who observed that the quality of nursing decisions, prescriptions and actions of clinicians, educators, managers and researchers will be optimized by the use of nursing research.

Resources outwith the place of employment

A range of local, regional, national and international research conferences provide an excellent means of further developing research knowledge and skill. These activities serve two major purposes. First, they give an insight into research, planning and data collection techniques. Second, they provide research based information relating to nursing practice, management and education. Creating a professional network with individuals engaged in research activity provides another useful means of learning about the subject. Having access to one or more of the many national libraries which carry a full range of research and other materials is another useful external resource. (See Chapter 10 for a discussion of these.)

Professional organizations such as the Royal College of Nursing have specialist societies, forums or interest groups. Membership of these specialist groups is available to members of the particular professional organization or may also be open to non-members. Research interest groups exist in a number of localities, these may be specific to nursing research or may have a more general focus. Short introductory courses relating to nursing research are now widely available. An introduction to nursing research now forms part of many post-registration courses. In addition to being taught the research process, students on these courses are now frequently asked to produce a research proposal or undertake a small research project, as part of the course work.

BECOMING A RESEARCHER

Although many nurses develop a sufficient level of knowledge and skill to enable them to undertake small projects in their place of work, and under the close supervision of an experienced researcher, a small number may wish to concentrate on that aspect of their career and become nurse researchers. It is not being suggested that clinicians, managers or teachers who perform a research function in addition to their normal work are making a lesser contribution than the specialist nurse researcher. Rather, it is recognized that a small number of nurses will go on to take a leadership role in relation to research and will become sufficiently skilled to enable them to lead research projects, supervise the research work of others, and choose to devote more of their time and energy in this area.

Many, but by no means all, research nurses study for a first degree in nursing or some related health care field. Others, have a degree level education in an area which is unrelated to health care. Such an education provides a firm academic foundation for acquiring a knowledge of the research base upon which research is founded. However, for those nurses who have a good grounding in clinical work, management or teaching, accompanied by an introduction to the research process in initial and subsequent education, studying for a basic degree might not be necessary.

The routes to a formal research education include part time or full time study for an MSc (Master of Science), MPhil (Master of Philosophy), and subsequently a PhD (Doctor of Philosophy) degree. Although many nurse researchers have studied for a PhD, others have learned their craft by one of a number of other means. These research degrees can either be part taught/research, or exclusively research based which is the usual practice in the UK. All are similar in that they require students to undertake a re-search study under the supervision of experienced researchers. Those which have no taught element, for example the PhD in the UK, may have a requirement that students read and understand a range of research textbooks and, if necessary, attend courses which will inform them of the range of research designs and methods.

Although a number of nurse researchers work on medium-or long-term contracts, others work on short-term (for example one year) contracts at the end of which they re-negotiate an extension or seek new employment. Nurse researchers are employed in nursing research units, government departments, institutes of higher education, such as universities and poly-technics, in some health boards, and on a variety of time-limited multi-disciplinary research projects. Career and employment opportunities for nurse researchers are undergoing a period of considerable expansion in the UK and in a number of other countries. Some nurse researchers have a combined research/clinical, research/management or research/teaching function. (See Bond (1984) for a discussion of the agencies supportive to nursing research generally, and to the nurse researcher in particular.)

IMPLEMENTING NURSING RESEARCH

One of the major reasons for the existence of nursing research is that it should (when appropriate) be implemented. The responsibility for imple-menting nursing research is shared by the nurse researcher and nurse clinicians, managers and educators who are potential consumers of the work. The researcher has a responsibility to produce a piece of work which has a relevance to nursing, and which contains specific references to the means by which it can be applied or otherwise used. At this point the role of the researcher in implementation is complete. The major responsibility for implementation lies with nurses to whom the research is addressed.

The implementation of research is not a clear and straightforward activity in which a well defined and discrete piece of research is implemented. More commonly, a piece of the research might be recognized as being of value in a particular setting. Alternatively, an amalgam of a number of studies might be combined for a particular purpose. Similarly, implementation of the research might result in a radical change in existing practice, modification of existing practice, or the substitution of a pre-existing method with something which is entirely different. Indeed, the outcome of a particular study might influence existing approaches to clinical practice, management or education by causing an individual or group of staff to construct new approaches which have been influenced by the research, but not specificially identified by it.

The relationship between research and development, and between research and change is an important one. Prior to the use of research in nursing, development and/or change frequently resulted from a 'common sense' approach. In the main, this approach to development and change has been relatively successful, although time consuming because of its trial and error basis. However, the use of scientifically based (research) approaches to development and change can considerably increase the possibility of success in terms of making the best kinds of alterations to existing practice, and in making conclusions with regard to the outcome.

Thus any change, whether or not it be research motivated, should have the outcome tested by the application of scientific principles. One way of doing this is, as far as is possible, to use existing research to make decisions regarding the kinds of changes which are necessary. By applying research principles to the implementation and evaluation of such change, one can be more certain regarding the desirability (or otherwise) of the outcome. In implementing research it is necessary that the nurse (or group of nurses concerned) should:

- Understand the general principles underlying the research process.
- Identify the specific problem which might be resolved by the implementation of research.
- Read and evaluate the research and non-research based literature on the subject.
- Select and/or adapt elements of existing research which are to be implemented.
- Discuss the problem area, the research literature, and possible methods of implementation with a nurse or some other person who has a knowledge of the subject area and of research.
- Discuss the problem area and associated research with colleagues and others who may be involved in its implementation. Unless full co-

operation is obtained from these other key people, it is probable that implementation will not be successful.

- Plan for the implementation of the research. Identify specific criteria against which success of implementation will be made.
- Collect pre-implementation data which will enable the measurement of success of implementation.
- Implement the research and collect data regarding its success.
- Evaluate the outcome of the implemented research and measure against the predetermined criteria for success.

The outcome of this type of research implementation will not only be of value to those doing it, it will be of considerable interest to researchers and others who are involved in this particular area of work. The author suggest that the question of publishing the outcome of such an activity should be seriously considered.

REFERENCES

Akinsanya, J. (1988) Complementary approaches. *Senior Nurse*, **8**(5), 20–2.
Bond, S. (1984) Agencies supportive to nursing research, in *The Research Process in Nursing* (ed. D.F.S. Cormack), Blackwell, London, pp. 21–9.
Cormack D.F.S. (1980) Obtaining access to data sources: an exploration of method, problems and possible solutions. *Journal of Advanced Nursing*, **5**, 357–70.
Cormack, D.F.S. (ed.) (1984) *The Research Process in Nursing*, Blackwell, London.
McFarlane of Llandaff (1984) Foreword in *The Research Process in Nursing* (ed. D.F.S. Cormack), Blackwell, London.
Pollock, L. and Tilley, S. (1988) Submitting for approval. *Senior Nurse*, **8**(5), 24–5.
Reid, N.G. and Boore, J.R.P. (1987) *Research Methods and Statistics in Health Care*, Edward Arnold, London.
Royal College of Nursing (1977) *Ethics Related to Research in Nursing*, Royal College of Nursing, London.
Wilson-Barnett, J. (1984) Gaining access to the research site, in *The Research Process in Nursing* (ed. D.F.S. Cormack) Blackwell, London.

FURTHER READING

Armitage, S. and Rees, C. (1988) Student projects: a practical framework. *Nurse Education Today*, **8**, 289–95.
Clark, E. (1987) Research awareness: its importance and practice. *The Professional Nurse*, **2**(11), 371–73.
Hunt, M. (1987) The process of translating research findings into nursing practice. *Journal of Advanced Nursing*, **12**, 101–10.
Mander, R. (1988) Encouraging students to be research minded. *Nurse Education Today*, **8**, 30–35.
Parahoo, K. and Reid, N. (1988) Research skills: Number 1. Getting started: The language of research. *Nursing Times*, **84**(39), 67–70.
    See subsequent four issues of the *Nursing Times* for the presentation of ideas and exercises designed to enable research skills development.

Sheehan, J. (1986) Nursing research in Britain: The state of the art. *Nurse Education Today*, **6**, 3–10.

Tierney, A., Closs, J., Atkinson, I. *et al.* (1988) On measurement and nursing research. *Nursing Times*, **84**(12), 55–8 (Occasional Paper).

Chapter 10

Reading the professional literature

DESMOND CORMACK
AND DAVID BENTON

For many years reading has been a major means of 'keeping up to date' for all professionals including nurses. Despite the current explosion in computer and video-based technology, the written word will continue to have an important part to play in the learning process. This need is reflected in the large numbers, national and international, of nursing and other health care journals which are currently being published. None of these journals would survive without an appropriate readership from library and individual subscriptions. Additionally, the boom in book publications which has taken place in the past ten or fifteen years testifies to the need for a greatly increased supply of published material in that form.

For many, the problem of what not to read is as much of a problem as deciding what to read. In short, because it is impossible to read all the material which is available we must become more selective in choice of materials.

In the past, it was fashionable to suggest that nurses were very poor at reading and that they failed to keep themselves fully aware of the contemporary literature (Boorer, 1969; Fisher and Strank, 1971). Although these criticisms may have been valid some years ago, nurses are undoubtedly developing a high level of skill in relation to reading appropriate and selected material. This development has had its roots in three areas: First, in the schools of nursing where the importance of the full use of the published literature has been emphasized; second, in work places where the availability of published materials, reports, written case studies and more detailed and informative patient reports is increasing; third, an increasing realization within the nursing profession that the present and future development of nursing as a profession, and of its individual members, is heavily dependent on the ability to make full use of written materials.

Although the profession generally is dependent on full use being made of the written word, it is the individual nurse who carries the responsibility for this task. There can be no doubt that reading forms the basis of a successful nursing education, is an important feature of all post-registration educational experiences, and is a fundamentally important part of the career development of every individual nurse. The differences between a nurse who is actively involved in reading, and one who is not, may be illustrated by two conversations which recently took place during which nurses were being interviewed for places on a post-registration course.

Example 1

Interviewer	'I'd like to turn to the ways in which you keep up to date with professional developments generally.'
Interviewee	'I attend conferences and study days, about four times per year, I also read as much as can.'
Interviewer	'I see . . . , what do you read?'
Interviewee	'The *Nursing Journal*.'
Interviewer	'How often do you read the *Nursing Journal*; do you buy it?'
Interviewee	'No, I don't buy it, I read it as often as I can in the hospital library.'
Interviewer	'What have you been reading about recently, has anything in particular caught your eye in the past few months?'
Interviewee	'I can't think of anything in particular.'
Interviewer	'Which issues have you seen discussed in the *Nursing Journal* in the past year?'
Interviewee	'I can't think of anything specific.'
Interviewer	'Have you bought and/or read a nursing textbook recently.'
Interviewee	'No, not since I finished my training twelve years ago.'

Fortunately, that kind of conversation in an interview is becoming increasingly rare. Contrast the second conversation in which the interviewee is able to demonstrate that she is involved in reading and, more importantly, is able to convince the interviewer that the material has been of value and has been remembered. Additionally, try and imagine the impact and influence which each of these interviews will have on the interviewee and interviewer respectively. While it is not being implied that the success or otherwise of the interview will be entirely dependent on the reading habits of the candidate, it is being implied that interviewers are paying much more attention to this skill in the correct belief that it is central to optimising the individual's level of functioning in whichever aspect of career development she chooses, and at whichever stage of career development she is at.

Example 2

Interviewer	'I'd like to turn to the ways in which you keep up to date with professional developments generally.'

Interviewee	'I attend conferences and study days about four times a year, I also read as much as I can.'
Interviewer	'I see . . . , what do you read?'
Interviewee	'The *Nursing Journal*.'
Interviewer	'How often do you read the *Nursing Journal*; do you buy it?'
Interviewee	'I don't buy it, I read it in the hospital library.'
Interviewer	'What have you been reading about recently, has anything in particular caught your eye?'
Interviewee	'Yes, a number of things, particularly the use of behavioural techniques in geriatric nursing, and the use of the nursing process.'
Interviewer	'Who has been writing about the nursing process recently?'
Interviewee	Names the author of a recent article on the nursing process and gives a brief summary of the content.
Interviewer	'Which issues have you seen raised in the *Nursing Journal* in the past year?'
Interviewee	Mentions two specific issues.
Interviewer	'What are your views on the first of these?'
Interviewee	Responds.
Interviewer	'Have you bought and/or read a nursing textbook recently?'
Interviewee	'I haven't bought one for sometime. I'm reading one at the moment, it's on geriatric nursing which is my specialty.'
Interviewer	'Why did you decide to read that particular book?'
Interviewee	'It was given an excellent review in the *Nursing Journal* last month.'

WHO SHOULD READ?

All professional nurses, of all grades, in all specialties, in all fields of nursing, whether administrators, researchers, teachers or clinicians, have a clear duty to be familiar with contemporary nursing literature (McLeod, 1988). This view, which is uncompromising, reflects the belief that professionalism and professional competence, are both heavily dependent on a knowledge of matters and issues which are outwith our immediate environment.

Not so many years ago a nurse who used a technique or procedure or process which was known by nurses in other parts of the country or world to be outdated or inadequate, may reasonably have used the excuse 'I just didn't know about that new method'. However, as is the case with other professions such as medicine, psychology, law and education, nursing professionals are expected to be fully aware of professional practice in other parts of the country, and of the world. The generally accepted means of achieving this awareness is via the professional literature.

WHY READ?

We all have different motivations and we will all read for different reasons. Where it is accepted that in such a personal issue as motivation it is not possible to identify all reasons, it is hoped that the majority of major stimuli for reading the professional literature are covered.

To improve patient care

If we accept that the prime function of the nursing profession is to cater for the needs of our clients, then reading the professional literature must be seen as a means of achieving improved standards of client care. This responsibility does not simply rest with clinicians but all nurses, administrators, educationalists and researchers alike. Often, due to the tendency towards specialization, the only opportunity available 'to make contact' with colleagues working in the same sphere is, in the first instance, by reading relevant material which may offer guidance in improving our own practice.

To learn

If we rely on personal experience and face-to-face contact with experts on our subject area, we will become aware of a very small percentage of the material which we need to know in order to function at our optimum level. For this reason books, journals and other forms of written material form a crucial part of any educational experiences. All teachers and subject experts realize that their knowledge of the subject is a small part of what is available. Thus, students, practitioners and teachers alike read to learn.

To keep up to date

In the past few decades all aspects of nursing have changed radically and rapidly. There is hardly an aspect of nursing education, practice, research or administration which has not been affected by rapid change, with nurses working in these areas experiencing real difficulty in keeping up to date.

While attendance at study days, conferences and seminars is a useful means of becoming aware of, and adapting to, change, the written word will remain an important means by which large numbers of people have fairly quick access to a means of keeping up to date and adapting accordingly.

Participation in debate

Almost all journals and publications from professional organizations and unions devote some space to debating current issues relating to the profession. The purpose of presenting these issues is two-fold: first, to present the views of the individual or organization; second, to stimulate public debate between groups and individuals which will, hopefully, result in those people contributing to the debate on issues. Thus, the written word can be used as a means by which the individual reader can contribute to the discussion of these issues which often radically effect his or her profession.

Course reading

Most, if not all, nursing courses contain a considerable amount of prescribed reading. In recent years it has become fashionable for course teachers to identify two kinds of reading: a short list of references which the student must read and a bibliography, or longer list of material with which the student should become generally familiar.

The authors' experience suggests that many such reading lists are overlong and contain many references which are of peripheral relevance to the subject being studied. Unless the reference lists are very short and sharp, then we are of the view that the teacher should help the student identify those items which are of most value and, more importantly, identify those chapters of often weighty texts which are of greatest relevance. Here, more than in any other aspect of reading, the importance of being selective is essential.

To satisfy curiosity

Perhaps the most important and rewarding reason for reading is to satisfy personal curiosity. Those who read because they want to, rather than because they have to, find the activity not only more stimulating, but also find the material more meaningful and more easily retained.

Reading for personal satisfaction is undoubtedly the most important means by which individual professional nurses maintain general awareness of professional development. For those who cannot, or prefer not to, attend formal educational courses then reading for the sheer pleasure of it, and to satisfy personal curiosity, will do much to continue their professional education in an 'informal' way.

WHEN SHOULD I READ?

Reading can make an important contribution to every part of professional development starting with the first day of pre-registration training and continuing until you decide to no longer play an active part in the nursing profession. Examples of when professional reading *may* no longer be important are when the decision has been taken to retire from nursing and to no longer play an active part in it.

WHERE TO READ

Although some reading will be done in the library, some personal time will have to be invested in reading at home. Nurses are increasingly regarding the investment of personal time in keeping up to date by reading as a natural part of personal and professional development. However, it is also being recognized by employers that they have an obligation to facilitate professional reading as part of the normal work process and commitment. Many places of work now have smalll libraries, journals and/or books on wards, facilities for the operation of journal clubs and a general expectation that nurses will make some use of reading materials during work time.

HOW DO I ORGANIZE READING?

Although actual reading is a very personal and individual matter, there are some general guidelines which may be of value in terms of organizing the task.

It is certainly necessary to read in a structured, organized and selective way which will make best use of time available for this activity. The sheer volume of available written material is far too large to 'dip into' in a random fashion in the hope that appropriate material will be discovered. Selecting appropriate material requires a general awareness of what is available. Second, it requires an ability to scan the available material and select only those which are of maximum importance.

SOURCES OF READING MATERIAL

Reading material for professional development can be found in nursing and other health care journals, newspapers and popular magazines, government and other national reports, items produced by unions and professional nursing organizations, textbooks, proceedings of conferences and employee produced reports and news sheets. Journals, as compared with textbooks, are certainly more up to date and varied in their content.

There are basically two kinds of journal which are directed specifically to the nursing profession: the 'general' journal which carries a wide cross-section of material. Examples are the *Nursing Times, American Journal of*

Nursing and the *Journal of Advanced Nursing*. Additionally, a wide range of specialist journals, such as those catering for geriatric, psychiatric and community nurses, are also available. Examples are *Journal of Gerontological Nursing*, *Journal of Psychosocial Nursing and Mental Health Services*, and *Journal of District Nursing*.

When thinking in terms of journal material, seriously consider the value of foreign journals (medical, social work, physiotherapy, and psychology ones for example) which are produced for health care professions other than nursing. The international nursing journal literature has a great deal to offer to nurses in countries other than those in which the journal was published. Similarly, the contents of non-nursing health care related journals often provide an invaluable source of material.

The question of whether or not to subscribe to a personal copy of a nursing journal is an important one. If there is access to a good nursing library which subscribes to a range of nursing journals then it is less necessary to obtain a personal copy. It is desirable to subscribe to at least one personal copy of a nursing journal either a specialist or general one. Having one's own copy of a journal increases motivation to both use it and become involved in the articles by way of writing letters to the journal and/or considering writing articles for publication. Furthermore, whilst borrowing journals from a library is certainly useful, experience has shown that if you subscribe to a journal you are unlikely to 'drift away' from the habit of reading and keeping up to date.

Another means of increasing the amount of literature available for personal use is for a small group of friends or nursing colleagues to purchase a small number of journals between them (one each) and circulate them between themselves. This may form the basis of a journal club which can be used to enable individuals to present summaries of materials which they have read relating to a certain topic.

Shelton (1988) described in detail the organization and management of a journal club which it was felt offered members the opportunity to develop skills in the reading, comprehension and evaluation of nursing literature. Additionally, members found that participation contributed to the development of their communication skills particularly the ability to discuss issues of concern in a group setting.

Library membership is an absolute necessity if you are to keep up to date with published materials. This aspect of personal, professional and career development cannot be over-emphasized. Almost all working nurses have reasonable access to a nearby hospital, college or nursing library. Additionally, those who work in large population centres will have access to university, college of education, central institution or polytechnic libraries. If none of these sources are available, or if they do not have the material that you require, access to certain national libraries can be sought (Table 10.1).

Table 10.1 National libraries

Library	Users and material available
Department of Health Alexander Fleming House Elephant and Castle London SE1 6BY Tel. 01 407 5522 Ext. 6363/6415	Open to all NHS employees but appointment is required. Holds an extensive international collection of material relating to health services. Photocopying available
Health Education Authority Health Promotion and Information Service 78 New Oxford Street London WC1A 1AH Tel. 01 631 0930	Open to the public. Wide selection of health education material. Photocopying and selective literature searching service available
Health Visitors' Association 50 Southwark Street London SE1 1UN Tel. 01 378 7255	Full service to HVA members, reference only to the public. Comprehensive selection of material on health visiting and allied subjects. Photocopying available
King's Fund Centre Library 126 Albert Street London NW1 7NF Tel. 01 267 6111	Open to the public without appointment. Extensive collection of material on health care, equipment and practice. Photocopying and literature search service
Northern Ireland Health and Social Services Library Queens University Institute of Clinical Science Grosvenor Road Belfast BT12 6BJ Tel. 0232 322043	Open to students and staff of Queens University and all health and social services staff throughout Northern Ireland. Comprehensive collection of material on all aspects of health and social sciences
Royal College of Midwives Library 15 Mansfield Street London W1 Tel. 01 580 6523	Open to RCM members, open to the public on request to the librarian. Extensive collection of material on midwifery and allied subjects. Manual and computerized literature search services available
Royal College of Nursing Library 20 Cavendish Square London W1M 0AB Tel. 01 409 3333 Ext. 345	Open to RCN members, non-members should contact the librarian. Holds the Steinberg collection of nursing research, and material on nursing and allied health subjects. Photocopying and bibliography service available
Scottish Health Service Centre Library Crewe Road South Edinburgh EH4 2LF Tel. 031 332 2335	Open to all Scottish Health Service employees. Comprehensive collection of material relating to all areas of health care and practice

(cont'd)

Table 10.1 (cont'd)

Library	Users and material available
Welsh National School of Medicine Library University of Wales School of Medicine Heathpark Cardiff CF4 4XN Tel. 0222 755944	Open to all students and staff of the University and for reference to all nurses. Collects material mainly on medicine, dentistry and nursing
Wellcome Institute for the History of Medicine Library 183 Euston Road London NW1 2BP Tel. 01 387 4477	Open to the public for research and reference only. Collection of material relating to the history of medicine and allied subjects

CHOOSING A LIBRARY

All libraries do not offer the same level of services (Cheung, 1988), this can vary considerably; the following is offered as a guideline with which to evaluate the quality of any nursing library which you may use.

1. Is there a comprehensive range of nursing textbooks which are up to date and cover all major (and minor) nursing specialties?
2. Is there a range of general and specialist national and international nursing journals? Additionally, is there a range of journals published primarily from non-nursing health care professionals? Ideally the library should have been subscribing to (and have back copies of) the journals for as long a period as possible.
3. A range of reference texts, including indexes and research abstracting systems is necessary.
4. An inter-library loan system is available in most libraries which enables an item not available in the library to be borrowed from other libraries. A good inter-library loan system will be inexpensive (if not free), will give a quick response to a request and will respond to almost any reasonable request.
5. Specialist libraries such as those found in universities which have a department of nursing, usually have a much larger number of librarians, some of whom may or may not be specialists in the subject of nursing literature. If such libraries do have a nursing specialist, then the help which that person can give to a reader is very considerable.
6. Most libraries will offer a photocopying service which will be reasonably priced and in some cases free. The more sophisticated service of telefax, a system where a copy of a document can be received (or sent)

instanteously on inter-library request is available at some libraries but can be more expensive.

7. Larger libraries will have a fully computerized catalogue which can be used for search as well as reservation and loan purposes, such a system is more efficient than manual methods.

8. The ability to conduct computerized literature searches is a real asset and can save hours of tedious searching through indexes. A good service will offer access to a number of the major index and abstract databases.

9. A variety of micro-fiche and micro-film reader machines should be available, ideally they should be able to produce a hard copy (paper printout) of any material required.

10. National libraries such as those administered by professional nursing organizations and government departments are accessible to the individual reader. Details about these libraries, and information about how to use them, should be available in your own library.

Having selected a library, using a library is not a skill which all trained nurses have (Childs and Walton, 1988). Although most recently trained staff will be familiar with how to use a small library, and some will be confident about using a major library, there are a number who have not been taught how to do so. If you have any reservations whatsoever about how to use the library, or feel reluctant to use it because of lack of confidence, approach the library staff and explain the position to them.

HOW CAN I FIND MATERIAL TO READ?

The biggest danger faced by most nurses who read the professional literature is the amount of information published. Only by being selective can optimal use of their reading time be ensured. Selective reading can be considered a cornerstone in career development.

Using the library catalogue

Every library has a catalogue of the material which it stocks and this can be thought of as a flexible index which can be used to find the piece of literature required. In some cases the library catalogue is a manual system using card indexes, in others a computer database. It is usual for there to be more than one catalogue. For example there is a catalogue for books, a catalogue for journals, and a catalogue for audiovisual materials.

In both computer and manual systems it is usual to access a book by either author or by subject. In the case of the computer system it may also be possible to look for material based on other criteria, such as, year of publication and title.

Books are stored in libraries by means of a subject classification scheme, that is all books relating to the same subject are kept together. There are many different types of subject classification schemes which are used to group books relating to particular subjects together. A number of classification systems are available each with advantages and disadvantages. However, there are two schemes which are commonly used in university, nursing and medical libraries:

1. *Dewey decimal classification scheme* (allows a numeric breakdown of all subjects from the general to the specific);
2. *National library of medicine classification scheme* (uses a combination of letters and numbers).

All libraries will have information on the classification system that they use, hence on joining ask the librarian for details and if possible get her to take you through looking for a book at least once.

In the case of libraries that use a manual system they will have manual card index catalogues, usually consisting of three distinct parts:

1. Author catalogue — a sequence of cards arranged alphabetically. Series entries are usually included as are joint authors and chairpersons of government committees.
2. Classification catalogue — these cards are sequenced according to the classification system in use within the library. The catalogue is an accurate copy of the order in which books appear on the shelves. This allows you to see at a glance what books the library has on a particular subject.
3. Subject index — this acts as an index to '2', enabling borrowers to locate specific subjects, either to check the classified catalogue or the shelves. Cards are arranged by subject, with each card noting the subject heading and corresponding classification code.

To look for a book on, for example, the nursing care of clients with senile dementia, would entail, in the case of the above manual system, reference to the subject index for both 'nursing care', and 'senile dementia' followed by examination of the shelves or the classification catalogue. Although the cross reference of the two sets of subject headings does work, such a system can be time consuming hence many libraries have opted to move their catalogue on to a computer database.

Computerized library catalogues offer a number of advantages over a manual system. First, the cross reference of subject headings can be carried out automatically, hence only those books on, in this case, nursing care of people suffering from senile dementia and not books on either nursing care or senile dementia will be found. Second, it identifies immediately whether (or not) a book is in stock, on loan, or reserved. Third it allows you to reserve books. Finally, it keeps much stricter control of the stock, recall letters are issued automatically when books are overdue.

Computerized systems are far more efficient and much more economical in terms of readers' time than manual systems. They allow the reader to use time reading rather than spend much time searching for material.

Indexes, abstracts and bibliographies

It is not financially possible for any one library to hold a stock of all books, periodicals, research reports, and other published material. Neither is it practical in terms of the space that such a mammoth collection would occupy. However, a good library will have the means to check exactly what has been published on any subject. The usual method used to determine this is by means of reference to indexes, abstracts, or bibliographies.

Indexes

The purpose of an index is to list all the material published in a defined group of journals on a particular subject. Indexes are usually produced monthly or quarterly and cumulated annually. Each journal article is listed under both author and subject(s). There are quite a few different indexes available and below there are examples of those applicable to nursing.

1. *Index medicus*, first published 1927, covers the whole field of clinical medicine and is published monthly with annual cumulations. The first issue of *Index Medicus* each year gives a listing of all journals indexed.
2. *International nursing index*, first published 1966, has an American bias which is reflected in subject terminology. Published quarterly.
3. *Cumulative index to nursing and allied health literature*, first published 1956, is a comprehensive index to the current periodical literature for nurses and allied health care professionals. It is published in five bi-monthly parts with the sixth bimonthly part being a cumulatively bound volume.

Abstracts

Abstracting journals summarize articles that have appeared in other journals. This can be a very useful service especially if you have only limited time available. Furthermore, unlike indexes which only provide the title, the reader can be absolutely sure of the articles content before obtaining a copy of the entire paper. Several abstracting journals exist, and those include:

1. *Nursing studies index*, which despite its name is an annotated (contains a short summary or abstract of the paper) guide to reported studies, research in progress, research methods and historical materials in periodicals, books and pamphlets, published in four volumes and covers the years 1900–1959.

2. *Nursing research abstracts*, is published quarterly and is based on the *index of nursing research data*. It is British in origin, has a primary focus in the nursing literature, and covers material published since 1977. A single volume of material for the years 1968–1976 is also available.
3. *Hospital abstracts*, was a monthly survey of the world literature and is prepared by the Department of Health and Social Security. It was first published in 1961 and covers the whole field of hospitals and their administration up until 1984.
4. *Health service abstracts*, has superseded *hospital abstracts*, and began publication in 1985. Published monthly, cumulative annual volumes are also available.

Bibliographies

Bibliographies are compilations of references found in books, periodicals and reports on some particular subject. Many national libraries regularly produce bibliographies which can act as valuable sources for a defined literature review. Various national libraries produce bibliographies which include:

1. *A bibliography of nursing literature*, published in two series by the Royal College of Nursing. The first series covers 1859–1960 and the second 1961–1970.
2. Scottish health service centre library publish regularly specialist bibliographies and reading lists (a type of current awareness service). Articles, reports, and books published are listed under various headings.

Several professional organizations as well as many college of nursing libraries provide a 'current awareness service'. This is a special type of bibliography that only consists of articles that are in the current issues of journals of recent publications an example of this type of service is *Nursing Bibliography*, which is published monthly by the Royal College of Nursing with annual cumulation since 1983. It presents a varied selection of material from books, periodicals, theses, reports and pamphlets. The Royal College of Midwives, and the Health Visitors Association also provide a current awareness service.

CONDUCTING A LITERATURE SEARCH

There is available to the professional nurse a vast source of reading material. Several tools are available to aid in the selection of specific material pertinent to a topic of interest, or for the purpose of professional development. However, such tools as the library catalogue, indexes, abstract-

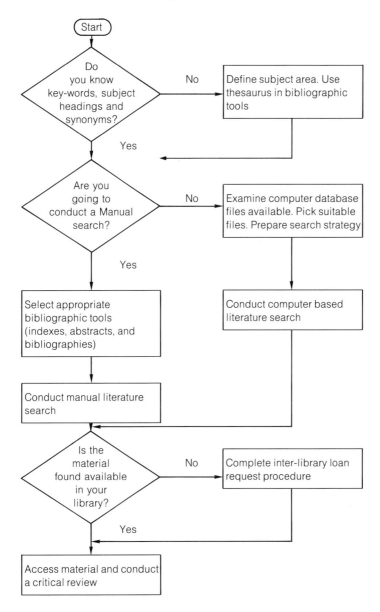

Figure10.1 Outline of the literature search process.

ing services and bibliographies must be used in a structured and logical manner if maximum benefit is to be derived.

Conducting a literature search efficiently is a skill professional nurses should develop if they are to be able to utilize the vast quantities of reading material available. The process is relatively mechanical, and can be easily learned providing the subject(s) of the search is known. Starting with the desire to find out about a specific subject, the approach outlined in Figure 10.1 will yield a list of reading material that can then be reviewed. Although some libraries may conduct a literature search for staff it is highly desirable that you are personally able to perform a literature search, since this may give valuable additional information about a topic, such as the volume of material available and the variety of sources.

When conducting the literature search there are two options which may be available, a manual search using the bibliographic tools already described, or a computerized literature search. Computerized literature searches use database files comparable to the manual tools. However, they are, on average, more up to date than their printed paper equivalents, and in addition to this, computerized literature searching has a number of other advantages:

1. Speed — millions of bibliographic references can be searched in seconds.
2. Flexibility — due to the interactive nature, computerized literature searches can be modified in light of the information you are retrieving.
3. Wide range of database files available — can be accessed via a telephone link to any location in the world.
4. Accessibility — unlike the printed equivalent which can be accessed via subject and author, computer databases can be searched by a variety of methods, for example, date of publication, journal title, or even a specific word in the article title.

In any system there are of course some disadvantages and on-line computerized literature searching is no exception, these include:

1. Coverage — this is a new technology and was not available prior to the early 1960s, hence it was rare to be able to search material published before that time. However, such is the demands for the service that most vendors are making earlier material available.
2. Technical problems — this can arise either with the computer or the telephone lines which can result in difficulties in being able to retrieve information.
3. Expense — in addition to purchasing the computer and the cost of telephone charges most database operators charge a yearly subscription and a fee in proportion to the amount of information you retrieve.
4. Need to be specific — if the search criteria are too vague, for example, keywords such as 'nursing' or authors such as 'Smith' then the number of references produced will be too large to be of value, and the cost will be excessive.

A number of companies provide on-line computer databases that can be used to conduct literature searches, each with its own procedures and language for formulating queries. To specify an efficient literature search strategy using a query language requires practice. Inefficient search strategies will result in increased telephone and access charges, hence it is common that most libraries will conduct computerized searches for you.

CONDUCTING A CRITICAL REVIEW OF THE LITERATURE

Whether you have conducted a literature search or are simply reading an article in your favourite professional journal, if you are to derive maximum benefit from the material you must review the article in a logical and critical manner, this is often referred to as conducting a 'critical review' of the material.

Most reading material follows a set pattern. The first step in the critical review is to recognize the format that has been used to write the material. By identifying the structure it is possible to first scan the article rapidly, knowing which sections to concentrate on and those to skip over, so as to assess whether or not the article is worth investing more of your time

Table 10.2 Key points in review of a research report

Title — is it concise and informative?

Abstract — (not always present) should summarize all major components of the study including the problem, hypothesis, methodology, major results and conclusions

Introduction — should give the rationale for the study and define the area to be investigated

Problem — the research problem should be clearly and concisely stated and any hypothesis should be in a form that allows it to be tested

Review of the literature — all cited literature should be relevant to the research problem and must be up to date. It must be organized in a logical manner and primary (original articles) should be reviewed as opposed to secondary sources (reports of other peoples reviews)

Methodology — should be clearly identified, with discussion of selection of any sample subjects, description of instruments especially their reliability and validity and also the specific research design used for conducting the study

Results — these must be presented in a clear, concise and readily understood form

Discussion — all results should be discussed in terms of their implications to the original problem, associated work conducted by other researchers may be used to compare and contrast the work undertaken in the study

Conclusions — conclusions should be justified in light of the results obtained and any flaws in the experiment identified and dealt with. Recommendations for future research may be made

---

in detailed reading. Perhaps the most valuable section of an article (if it exists) is the abstract, for this should include all the vital information about the paper — always read the abstract in full. The next step is to identify all headings and subheadings, thus allowing you to focus on those parts of greatest interest to you. Generally speaking, the introduction and conclusion should give, in the absence of an abstract, enough information as to whether a detailed review would be of value.

Certain types of article for example, the research report, follow a standard pattern, and when reviewing such articles it is important to identify a number of key points, these are summarized in Table 10.2.

KEEPING TRACK OF YOUR READING

Reading the professional literature is only of real value if you can quickly and accurately recall the material. Several different ways of keeping track of the professional literature are available. Tyznik (1983) suggested that articles should be coded using the International Classification of Diseases, 9th Revision, Clinical Modification (ICD-9-CM), then filed under the appropriate code in a series of folders.

Emerson and Jackson (1982) described the use of a 'marginal punch sort card system'. This involved the use of index cards with a series of holes cut into the margins. Articles were categorized and the position of the holes determine the category to which an article belonged. The holes could then be used at a later date to retrieve articles on a specific category or by repeated selection on a number of categories.

All nurses have access to the requirements for the system described by Emerson and Jackson since it is based upon 4 × 6 in pieces of card. The degree of flexibility in sorting references approaches that of some of the more basic computer systems. For example, all cards storing information related to one particular subject can be extracted, then they can be further sorted by a further criterion, perhaps by journal.

With the advent of the personal computer and low cost database software

Table 10.3 Information required to be stored on a reviewed publication

Authors:–	Publication date:–	
Article title:–		
Book title:–		
Journal:–		
Vol. and part No:–	Page nos:–	Active:–
Editors:–		
Publication place:–	Publisher:–	
Key words:–		
Abstract:–		

packages another option open for the storage of references is available. A reference database can be thought of as a home based library catalogue which can offer the rapid, efficient storage and retrieval as well as printing of references. Typically the sort of information that should be recorded can be seen in Table 10.3.

Most of the headings in Table 10.3 are self-explanatory, but the heading 'Active' is unique to a computer based reference storage system. This is what is known as a 'Logical Category', it has the value 'true' or 'false' and it is used to indicate that the reference is being used for an active reference list. The system can then be asked to output a copy of the reference list by simply identifying those references for which the value of 'Active' is 'true'. This gives the computer system the added advantages of reducing transcription errors, and reduction in typing time.

The computerized storage of information on articles which you have reviewed offers a great deal of flexibility in the manner in which references can be recalled. As many headings as you wish can be used, either individually or in combination, to recall material. This type of system also can be used to determine whether or not to continue subscribing to a particular journal, since it is possible to extract a profile of the number of articles you have references from that journal over a certain time period. If you find that you are no longer regularly referencing material, from a journal you subscribe to, it may be time to consider changing your subscription to an alternative publication.

REFERENCES

Boorer, D. (1969) Nurses who do not read. *Nursing Times*, **65**(31), 984–5.

Cheung, P. (1988) Library and Information Services in a Health Authority. *Nurse Education Today*, **8**(6), 364–5.

Childs, S. and Walton, G. (1988) Newcastle Upon Tyne Polytechnic Library and Information Services to Nurses in Northern Regional Health Authority. *Nurse Education Today*, **8**(6), 365–6.

Emerson, S.C. and Jackson, M.M. (1982) Organize your references. *Nursing Administration*, **13**(6), 33–7.

Fisher, R.F. and Strank, R.A. (1971) Investigation into the reading habits of qualified nurses. *Nursing Times*, **67**(8), 245–7.

McLeod, F.G. (1988) Towards coherence in the education of nursing students in information skills. *NBS News Update*, December 1988, 3.

Shelton, S.E. (1988) Keeping pace with nursing literature through a professional gerontological nursing journal club. *Journal of Gerontological Nursing*, **14**(11), 26–8.

Tyznik, J.W. (1983) Taming the medical literature 'monster'. *Postgraduate Medicine*, **74**(1), 77–80.

Chapter 11

Information technology

DAVID, BENTON

Man is currently living in an increasingly information-dependent society. Consequently, from the cradle to the grave, new technology has a profound effect upon us all. Daily, information is added to the sum total of our knowledge, knowledge that we are required to locate, use and pass on to our descendants. Although this is a rather macroscopic view, it does reflect the fact that all individuals, including nurses, are required to use increasing numbers of technological devices in their everyday work.

The term 'information technology' is regularly used by both professionals and lay people, often with little thought as to its meaning. Essentially, information technology refers to the amalgamation of the storage and processing powers of computers, with the ability to distribute information either locally, nationally, or internationally via various communications networks, for example, by telephone, or by satellite.

The documentation of health care generates large amounts of information, consequently nurses who will be practising into the next century will require information technology skills as part of their professional repertoire.

COMPUTER LITERACY

It is not necessary for users to understand the means by which data manipulation takes place. However, it is essential that the underlying concepts, capabilities and limitations of the various systems are understood. For example, many people drive cars but are unable to perform more than the simplest of maintenance tasks. This does not prevent use of the vehicle to get from point A to point B, provided they have the necessary knowledge and skills to operate the car. Similarly, nurses who are computer literate, that is those who have basic knowledge of computers and skills in their use, are able to use computers as useful tools in the efficient development of nursing practises.

Nationally, a call for the inclusion of computer literacy in the core syllabus of all nursing students was made by the Royal College of Nursing (1984) in their recommendations for nursing education through the next decade. In that report, a six-month common training for all nurses was suggested. During this time students would be exposed to a foundation course which would equip them with the basic skills, knowledge, attitudes and nursing concepts essential to all nurses. Computer literacy was identified and included as one of the common elements required for all nurses.

The National Board for Nursing, Midwifery and Health Visiting for Scotland (1985) issued guidelines for continuing education in the form of Professional Studies One and Two. Close examination of Professional Studies One reveals that, amongst the options for study, is a module on computer studies and its relation to nursing. More recently, the means of introducing health care professionals to information technology has been examined by the World Health Organization (1986). On discovering a lack of knowledge and skills amongst health workers in the implementation and use of new technology, they identified the need for carefully structured educational programmes in health care computing so as to produce computer-literate health professionals, instead of having to rely on information technologists with no health care knowledge.

Presently, Britain is behind some parts of Europe in the education of nurses in computer literacy. However, despite this, the British Computer Society (BCS) has a small support group, BCS nursing specialist group,* which provides regular newsletters to its members on information technology and its application to nursing. The group has also been responsible for the publication of a regular supplement, *Computers In Nursing News* (CINNEWS) in one of the national nursing magazines (*Nursing Times*). The supplement deals with many basic issues relating to the introduction and implementation of computers in all areas of nursing practice. Internationally, Townsend and Norman (1985) reported that Dutch nurse managers had access to a four-month day-release course at the University of Leiden aimed at providing them with enough information to enable them to contribute positively in the process of acquisition and implementation of new information technology systems for nurses.

In Sweden, Gerdin-Jelger (1984) commented that the role of computers in nursing was changing since computer applications had moved towards the care level. This prompted computer literacy and health care informatics (the scientific study and application of information technology) to be included in the training syllabus of nurses in that country.

At present, few nurses understand the basic functions of computer systems and hence are (wrongly) reluctant to use them. Grobe (1984) expressed the view that nurses 'feared' computers due to their lack of basic knowledge, familiarity and understanding of the machines, and their

---

* Further information can be obtained from the British Computer Society Headquarters, 13 Mansfield Street, London W1M 0BP.

application to health care. Hoy (1987) highlighted another particularly important point which can impede the successful implementation and use of new technology, namely that some staff have unrealistic perceptions of computers and their capabilities, greatly overestimating the power of the machine and imagining that it will be able to solve all their problems.

Thomas (1988) recognized that the amount of knowledge and skills required to use new technology will vary depending on the nurse's position and responsibilities within the organization. A modular approach to training was advocated, with all nurses receiving rudimentary training in the application of new technology as part of their pre-registration education. Those individuals who are required to take decisions with regards selection of equipment and development of information technology strategies, would require more advanced knowledge and skills training. In brief, the numbers of nurses and the degree of skills required can be represented in graphic form (Figure 11.1).

From Figure 11.1 it can be seen that a number of modules (**a**–**e**) might be required. Although five modules are shown it is not intended that this should be prescriptive since the exact content and number of modules

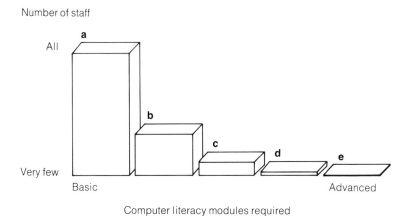

Figure 11.1   Numbers of staff and the extent of computer literacy required. **a**, All staff spend 2–3 hours finding out what a computer looks like, how it is switched on and how to communicate with it (keyboard skills); **b**, Ward managers require skills sufficient to teach their staff how to use the specific pieces of equipment in their own wards; **c**, Section managers require knowledge to co-ordinate services across a number of wards and suggest improvements to the system; **d**, Staff at unit and district level require sufficient knowledge and skills to take strategic planning decisions with regards the purchase of equipment and methods of implementation; **e**, Very few staff will be required to liaise with computer experts for the purpose of developing new systems. They will require sufficient levels of knowledge to be actively involved in the design of software.

required to cater for the computer literacy needs of staff is outwith the focus of this chapter. Nevertheless, it would be envisaged that module **a** would form part of the core syllabus of pre-registration training and act as an introduction to computers and their use. This would equip staff to use existing systems. Those staff with additional responsibilities for the introduction, implementation, development, or purchasing of systems would require further training (modules **b–e**).

Although computers can be applied to a variety of situations, most systems are essentially manipulators of information. The manner in which data are manipulated depends essentially upon the underlying programme structure. Three basic programme structures are commonly found; word-processors that allow the production of perfect documents or personalization of standard letters; databases that store vast amounts of information which can be sorted and later retrieved in flexible formats; and spreadsheets that enable the manipulation of mainly numerical data, allowing a variety of options to be appraised based on alternative strategies posed by the user. Due to the widespread application of these core structures, basic knowledge of the capabilities and limitations of all three are essential if nurses are to be able to use systems which utilize these approaches.

Recent government legislation in the form of the Data Protection Act has been issued regarding the rights of access by individuals to data kept about them (Her Majesty's Stationery Office, 1984). Modifications, which effectively limits access by patients to their medical records, if it is judged to be potentially detrimental to their treatment, have been made (Common Services Agency, 1987). If nurses are to keep within the law, then the importance of data security and the rights of access must be appreciated.

A series of eight guideline booklets* on the Data Protection act have been published and are available free of charge. Perhaps the most useful booklet for nurses is guideline booklet No. 1 '*Introduction to the Act*' (Data Protection Registrar, 1987). The introductory booklet gives rudimentary details of the Act and clarifies the point that the Act only applies to information that is processed by computers, and relates only to individuals who are living.

APPLICATIONS OF COMPUTERS IN NURSING

To date, nursing has seen a wide variety of computer applications implemented into health care, many of which have direct effects on the role and function of the nurse. However, developments have been rather uncoordinated and generally these have been the result of individuals or groups

---

* Available from Office of the Data Protection Registrar, Springfield House, Water Lane, Wilmslow, Cheshire, SK9 5AX.

with computer skills applying their knowledge to specific (often localized) problems. Hence it is unusual to see all applications being used in any one health care area, or for any one application to be used throughout the UK. Nevertheless the likelihood exists that as experimental systems are evaluated then some, if not all, will be applied more widely.

A difficulty with any computer system is one of categorization. Systems tend to develop and integrate additional applications as information, staff and patient needs are identified. This has resulted in few, if any, applications standing alone, hence the categorization that follows in this chapter is rather artificial since most systems will cater for a number of applications and not just one in isolation.

Patient administration systems

Patient Administration Systems (PAS) are perhaps one of the most common forms of new technology that has been introduced into health care. Initially they tended to be used almost exclusively within the confines of the medical records department, and provided information to general management on such topics as hospital utilization, consultant outpatient workloads and waiting list statistics.

Problems arose in the early development of PAS due to difficulties in deciding on the types of information that should be gathered about patients. Körner (Department of Health and Social Security, 1982) examined this issue and produced a minimum data set for a variety of specialist areas. These data sets ensure that there is at least a minimum level of compatible and comparable data between different health boards and health authorities. The need for consistency between health boards/authorities has resulted in joint developments of systems which has contributed to the more widespread implementation of PAS.

The Körner data set can be used to great advantage by the nurse in the ward, since it is no longer necessary to duplicate information gathering activities which have already taken place in other areas of the hospital. Nurses can be released from a great deal of form filling activity since name, address, and history can all be recalled from the data file and printed out when requested from terminals in the ward. Additionally, the information is always legible. Unlike existing manual file systems information can be available in more than one location at any time. Files are no longer unavailable due to being in transit from ward to ward. Finally, due to standard computer operating procedures copies of the information are made on a regular basis, hence no files can go missing.

Royce (1987) identified that PAS can function 24 hours a day, seven days a week and, in addition, can integrate information from many sources.

These factors led him to believe that PAS would rapidly develop into a true multi-user system with all health care professionals making contributions to the patient data file.

PAS holds information centrally that can be distributed and accessed at many locations. This can cause concern to patients who may seek assurance as to the security of the data that they provide. Furthermore, patients may ask about the system and how it works. Both these issues can cause difficulties for staff who are ill prepared to deal with them. It is therefore considered essential that adequate training be provided so as to equip nurses with the knowledge and skills to deal with patient enquiries.

The security of PAS can be achieved by a variety of methods. Terminals can be located in physically secure areas, with only authorized personnel getting access. Although practical for medical records departments, ward-based systems require more flexible security measures. Special keys to turn on the system or unlock the keyboard may be used by the nurse in charge. However, the most commonly used means of controlling security access is by issuing passwords to staff. Different levels of access can be controlled, for example nursing staff may access and modify the nursing record, but only medical staff can access and modify the drug prescription sheet.

Patient care planning

A natural extension of PAS is to incorporate the documentation of day-to-day care into the system so as to enable the provision of a specific daily nursing care plan. Harrow (1988) identified several advantages of such a system which has been in operation for over ten years at Ninewells Hospital Dundee. It was noted that, prior to implementation, staff had been struggling to document care. Examination of patient data recording sheets showed that 50% of the required information was omitted. After implementation of the computerized system, patient data forms were found to be fully completed. Another benefit is the time saving that resulted due to the ability to search the patient record automatically using a simple interrogation facility which, for example, allows the nurse by use of certain verbs to 'FIND', 'GET' or 'PRINT' the required information. Furthermore, Cook (1982) noted that the reduction in nurses' time spent on administrative and routine clerical tasks, now carried out by the computer, had freed nurses, allowing them to provide more direct patient care.

One difficulty of computerized patient care planning was highlighted by Gebhardt (1983), in that problems can exist in the quality of input data. This may be caused by typographic errors; however, system interfaces that utilize menu selection can help to reduce such problems by making data entry easier and more accurate (Figure 11.2).

```
┌─────────────────────────────────────────────┐
│          S Y S T E M   S E L E C T I O N      │
│                                               │
│                  Married                      │
│                  Divorced                     │
│                  Single                       │
│                                               │
├─────────────────────────────────────────────┤
│ Choose option by pressing highlighted letter  │
└─────────────────────────────────────────────┘
```

Figure 11.2 Example menu selection system.

Patient monitoring

The use of new technology in patient monitoring, that is where vital signs such as pulse, respiration rate and temperature are recorded by machines, has been in existence for some time. These systems were introduced into the high-tech nursing areas such as coronary care and intensive care units.

Initially the systems were used to calculate and regulate very precisely the flow rate of infusions, or were used to sound alarms when pre-set conditions (decided by the nurse) occurred, for example, pulse rate or respiration rate above or below specific levels. With developments in new technology, and since the cost of equipment in real terms has dropped, monitoring systems are now being used more widely throughout hospitals.

Computerized systems have now the ability to analyse the data they gather. In the case of electrocardiography, monitoring equipment is able to recognize abnormal rhythms and record the episode. Staff can then be alerted, all without the need for manual intervention. These records can become the basis of discussion material, comparing these episodes with the treatment regime for the patient (Beckmann *et al.*, 1981). Computerized approaches to patient monitoring free nurses from the technician role of watching machinery in the high-tech areas of intensive and coronary care units (Ball and Hannah, 1984). However, this does require nurses to have high levels of knowledge and confidence in using such equipment. Although nurses with advanced skills, and those who have completed intensive therapy courses, already have experience in using the equipment, many nurses in ward areas are less fortunate. McMenemin *et al.* (1987) concluded that unless staff are familiar with the implementation and use of these systems the widespread use will be inhibited.

Patient assessment

Various tests have been developed over the years, that enables a number of characteristics to be assessed, based on clients' responses to questionnaires, personality inventories and other assessment scales.

Generally, they are computerized versions of paper and pencil tests that have been validated and used for many years. However, the computer allows instant scoring which enables the therapist to assess the effects of interventions without having to complete the usual lengthy and tedious process of manual scoring.

Research has shown that certain client groups prefer using computers for testing. Skinner and Allen (1983) demonstrated that the accuracy of the information gathered was much higher when computers were used. They found that clients were more open and honest with the computer, compared with face-to-face interview. Investigation of the differences between the two methods of data collection revealed that clients saw the computer as less judgemental, resulting in more accurate information.

Several studies have reported the use of computers for patient assessment, but they tend to be conducted by medical staff and psychologists. There is, however, evidence that as systems become more widely utilized, nursing staff are given the responsibility for data collection and evaluation (Hunter, 1987).

Administrative uses

New technology has been used for years as a means of reducing the administrative workloads of professionals. Programmes are available that can reduce the burden of routine administrative tasks, hence it is not surprising to see the rapid introduction of many systems in the area of nurse administration.

Stonier (1988) stated that the most valuable resource within the National Health Service is the workforce. Within any organization employing large numbers of staff there is a need to keep accurate and up to date personnel records.

It is common for monthly 'starters' and 'leavers' reports to be required so as to enable the control of hospital establishment figures. Bell and Catchpole (1984) described how a personnel system was set up and implemented, which catered for these requirements. A standard database package was used to store the necessary information and generate the required monthly reports.

It was recognized that the production of such a system is one thing, but its implementation by managers is another. To achieve system usage, it had to be seen as credible and usable by all managers, offering them ways of managing the service in a more efficient manner. Education and training was seen to be the key to the successful implementation.

Several authors have utilized computer systems for the production of duty rotas and the monitoring of sickness patterns (Squire, 1982; Darley, 1983; Canter, 1984; and Moores and Murphy, 1984). In these cases individual programmes, written to perform one specified task, as opposed to off-the-shelf packages, such as spreadsheets that could be modified to fulfil a variety of tasks, were used. This required the authoring and coding, as well as debugging, of the programmes. All three activities, particularly debugging, which is the process of removing errors in the programme and ensuring that it performs the tasks required, are highly specialized and would normally be performed by computer programmers. Few nurses have these skills and even fewer have the time to carry out such work. However, if managers are conversant with the technology and can communicate effectively their needs to the appropriate expert, then team approaches to problem solving can be utilized.

New technology, primarily installed for other functions, can be utilized by managers as a means of facilitating communication with ward staff. Berrill (1986) describes how a PAS was modified to support other options. Viewdata type screen output, which is similar in format to the screens available on CEEFAX and ORACLE, was available that could notify staff of urgent messages. When staff turned on the terminal for PAS, messages appeared before the main system was accessed. Staff could not bypass the screens, and messages added to the system after the terminal had been switched on used an additional facility to notify staff of the new urgent message. In addition to messages, the system was also used for storing a copy of the hospital procedures manual. This had the advantage that, once amendments were made to the master copy, all subsequent access to the onscreen procedures were accurate and up to date. No longer had staff to search for the manual since it was available via the terminal located in the ward. Copies of the required procedure could be made by using the ward printer.

Decision support systems

With the ever increasing volume of information nurses are required to gather and organize, it is hardly surprising that computers are now beginning to be introduced which support the decision-making process. If resources are limited and a decision is to be made, then efficient use of the information, getting the priorities right, is required. Over the last decade in this country, since the introduction of the nursing process, nurses are looking at problems in a much more logical manner. Cause and effect relationships are being identified and evaluation of outcomes is an integral part of this approach. Often, decision criteria can be identified and used to improve care.

One example of such a system is described by Hyslop and Jones (1986) who developed over 40 criteria that enable the accurate assessment of pressure sore development risk. Data are required on a number of criteria and, based on nurses' responses to various questions, the system objectively rates the client for pressure sore development risk. The nurse can then allocate the resources based on this and other information appropriate to the clients' needs.

Some nurses are concerned that these systems will 'take over' the decision-making process, but there is no evidence from the nursing profession to support this statement. Clancy (1979) on reviewing the use of an antibiotic prescribing aid used by the medical profession, found that the system facilitated more rapid decision making by doctors. The system did not take over, since doctors were free to either accept or reject the advice given.

The major problem with decision support systems is the difficulty in identifying and formalizing the criteria that nurses currently use to make decisions. This is not a problem unique to the nursing profession, since a completely new science, knowledge engineering, has evolved which tackles the whole issue of knowledge representation and the generation of expert systems.

Computer-supported education

Over the last ten years there has been a rapid growth in interest in the use of computers as a means of educating nursing staff. A recent report by the National Board for Nursing, Midwifery and Health Visiting for Scotland (1987) gave a detailed history of the development of a nationally co-ordinated approach to the production of high quality educational programmes which can be run on a microcomputer. A wide variety of topics have been covered and there are plans for many more. These packages, which have been evaluated by the majority of those colleges of nursing that have the necessary equipment, have been well received and are considered a success.

Until recently, the educational effects of computer-assisted learning had not been fully evaluated. However, some studies have now been published which indicate that computers can make an effective and efficient contribution to pre- and post-registration education.

Benton (1988) reported that a group of trained psychiatric nurses could learn significantly more from a computer programme, in less time, than a group that used standard lecture/discussion methods to study the same subject. The nurses in the study identified a number of advantages of using the system:

1. Staff could learn at their own pace;
2. Privacy, the ability to make mistakes without ridicule;
3. The ability to receive remedial information when staff answered a question wrongly;
4. The system was easy to use;
5. Reinforcement was given after each correct answer;

6. Active, as opposed to passive, learning;
7. Motivational (some staff took part in their own time);
8. Demands staff's attention;
9. Flexibility, can be used when staff want to learn or when it is convenient.

There were, however, some disadvantages and these included:

1. Ergonomics of the man/machine interface. For example some people found the chair uncomfortable for prolonged use;
2. Having to use a typewriter keyboard;
3. Anxiety at having to use a computer;
4. Not being able to backtrack through the presented material.

A study conducted by Norman (1988) of advanced procedural knowledge in the administration of intravenous medications also reported favourable results. Staff who used the package demonstrated improved knowledge achievement scores and found it '...stimulating...', '...enjoyable...', and '...absorbing...'.

Since it would appear that computers can be used successfully in the education of staff, and with the increased availability of equipment, it may be possible in the future to incorporate educational packages on how to use the systems as part of the overall design of new technology for nurses in the future.

Word processor applications

Word processors are a type of computer programme which allow the user to manipulate text until the perfect document is produced. Unlike conventional typewritten material there is no need to retype correct passages, words, or sentences. Paragraphs or chapters can be added, removed, moved or modified with the greatest of ease. The final document can then be printed out when the author is satisfied with the material. Many systems offer advanced features such as automatic spelling checking, indexing and type setting, or facilities like thesaurus and self help. Some systems can, in addition to the word processing features, provide a typing tutorial that will teach the user to touch type.

Most systems offer a merging facility whereby standard letters can be merged with personal details, thus resulting in individualized copies of the letter. This can be very useful to nurse researchers who are conducting survey type studies, since letters can be personally addressed to the subjects concerned.

Once data are gathered, the word processor can then be used to write a research report, article, or thesis. McDonald (1984) identified, in addition to the features already discussed, that a word processed thesis was less expensive to produce, particularly if several drafts were required, than one produced by standard typewritten methods. Although it may be considered most appropriate to include word processors under 'Research Applications' they have much wider use since they can also be used to write articles, nursing notes or any application that requires the recording of written textual material. Advanced word processors also allow the user to merge screens of (already prepared) graphics, such as pie or bar charts, into the text of reports.

A recent publication by Catchpole *et al.* (1987) highlighted the flexibility of a handheld keyboard operated data recording system, a simple form of word processor, which was used by district nurses and health visitors to make notes on their client visits. At the end of each day, or when they returned to their base, the information was transferred to their main record-keeping computer. In evaluating the handheld data recorders, nurses found the system easy to use and faster than paper methods of note taking. In addition, due to the printed output, relief nurses were able to easily read colleagues' records, hence improving continuity of care.

Research applications

Computers have been used for many years as a tool to aid researchers with various tasks. The data manipulation capabilities of the computer can be exploited by nurse researchers in several ways.

Word processors can be a very useful tool to the nurse researcher. Reports, articles, books and research theses can all be produced with much greater ease due to the flexibility of redrafting offered by this approach as opposed to traditional typewritten methods.

Statistical analysis is often an essential part of any research study. Analysis of data can be tedious, repetitive and prone to errors if manual means of computation are used. Many software packages are available which can make light work of data that would have taken hours, days, or even weeks to analyse by hand.

Database systems are another area that can be used by the nurse undertaking research. As more and more data are held on computers, research nurses will turn to databases as a source of historical information for analysis. Already, many researchers use the capabilities of database interrogation to conduct literature searches.

Smith (1988) reported that approximately quarter of a million articles are published in the health sciences every year. With such a large number of articles being produced, it is extremely difficult for any individual to access and review all material pertinent to a research topic. One solution to this problem is electronic bibliographic searching. Searches can be conducted by any of a number of identifying characteristics or fields, for example by author, year, publication, or key words in the abstract or title. However, one major drawback of any computer database search is that if search criteria are posed in a loose non-specific way, the resulting search will yield hundreds or even thousands of articles. Many of these articles may only be loosely related to the search criteria. If the key words used are too specific, the resulting articles are all applicable, but valuable material may be missed. Nurses must therefore strike an appropriate balance between the two extremes (for a full discussion see Chapter 10).

An example of a computer literature search for articles related to the evaluation of computer-assisted instruction methods is shown in Table 11.1. The search lists the number of articles found when each of the key words are specified. When these key words are combined by asking the computer to identify only articles that relate to all the criteria a much smaller but manageable set of articles is produced.

The search illustrated in Table 11.1 was performed using the ERIC (Educational Resource Information Centre) database and took 1 minute 42 seconds, at a cost of 4 American dollars. A simple request for a print-out of the titles, authors, sources and abstracts (at point*) yielded a bibliography of material that was up to date, applicable to the research topic and inexpensive both in terms of cost and researchers time.

Over the past ten years, increasing numbers of nurses have been trained in research methods, many of whom have been exposed to the advantages of employing the use of information technology as tools in conducting research. As nurse training under the development of the United Kingdom Central Council for Nursing, Midwifery and Health Visiting's (1987) Project 2000 proposals move towards a more research-based education, even more nurses will be given the opportunity to develop research skills and hence access to computers.

Table 11.1 Sample dialogue of computerized literature search

FIND 'Computer'	24 357 articles on file
FIND 'Assisted'	9689 articles on file
FIND 'Instruction'	107 485 articles on file
FIND 'Computer' WITH 'Assisted' WITH 'Instruction' (string 1)	7907 articles on file
FIND 'Evaluation'	95 141 articles on file
FIND 'Methods'	91 337 articles on file
FIND 'Evaluation' WITH 'Methods' (string 2)	4948 articles on file
FIND string 1 WITH string 2	159 articles on file
(i.e. Computer assisted learning evaluation methods)	
PRINT string 1 WITH string 2*	
(gives a paper print-out of the references)	

Communication aids

New technology can be used to significantly enhance the quality of life of both physically and mentally disabled individuals. Before the advent of cheap and reliable microcomputers, many patients were unable to achieve their full potential due to limitations placed upon them by their disabilities. Individuals who are quadriplegic and also unable to speak, can, by the use of micro technology, become mobile and able to communicate, using systems that free them from their physical and mental difficulties. Patients can, by the use of specially designed and adapted keyboards, communicate effectively both in written and, by the use of voice synthesizers, in verbal form.

Generally speaking, professionals other than nurses are responsible for the assessment, adaptation and development of such aids. Nevertheless, if nurses are to be responsible for the maximization of patients' capabilities then they need knowledge of the equipment available.

Supplies ordering

Any nurse who has had to complete the weekly stores requisition knows how tedious and time consuming it can be. First, having to check what is in stock, then trying to recall which department supplies the item. If this is not bad enough, how infuriating it is to find out a few days later when the stores are delivered, that the very items required most urgently are out of stock.

Large manufacturing organizations have for years had sophisticated stock control systems. When a predetermined balance is reached, an order invoice is issued to the supplier so that the new stock arrives before the current stock is exhausted. New technology has made this process for some companies fully automatic.

Hospitals with ward-based terminals could use them to order supplies direct from the stores. The systems could be automated so that all the nurse has to do is give details of the balance remaining on the ward, and the system could do the rest. If an item was unavailable then she would be notified immediately.

Ashton (1983) described a system that took the automatic ordering of supplies one step further. In this case the supply in question was the pharmacy drug order. Medical staff had to record their prescription direct on to a computer system. This had several advantages: prescriptions were legible; drugs were always prescribed using the approved names; checks with the patient administration system that the client did not have any allergies to the drug were made; any potential drug interaction effects with concurrent medication were identified; stock balances were checked and the amount required ordered from pharmacy. This system, while reducing the administrative workload, also provides a safer service to the patient.

CONCLUSIONS

As nurses develop understanding of new technology then inevitably new applications will be identified. If these systems are designed with appropriate nursing input, then many potential problems can be avoided. To enable this level of input, more advanced skills will be needed. Elementary knowledge and skills in systems analysis and design will be required by certain nurses (Adams, 1986).

Technology offers the nursing profession many attractive advantages, both in terms of reducing administrative workload and improving direct client care. Those nurses with knowledge and skills in the use of information technology will have the power and influence not only to direct their own future development, but also that of the profession. Nurses without these skills will be severely disadvantaged and, through their lack of knowledge, may resist the implementation of systems as an expression of their anxiety and fears of the new technology.

Computers are already used in all areas of nursing practice, and as the numbers of these devices increase, the demands for well-informed nurses to use the systems will also increase. Computer literacy is seen as being required as an urgent and essential addition to the nursing curriculum.

When these issues are dealt with, the nurses being trained will be well equipped and prepared to deal with the new technology challenges beyond the year 2000. With nurse educationalists about to review the curriculum in preparation for implementation of Project 2000 (United Kingdom Central Council for Nursing, Midwifery and Health Visiting, 1987), an ideal opportunity exists to integrate computer literacy into pre-registration education, hence taking steps to safeguard the development of the nursing profession into the next century.

The increase in the use of information technology offers nurses further opportunities for career development. New dimensions, in the form of computer literacy, can be added to the nurse's role. Furthermore, many health boards and authorities have created or will create in the near future, posts specifically for the purpose of integrating new technology into nursing practice. Nurses must be prepared to take full advantage of these opportunities. That they will have the motivation and the ability to meet this new challenge is beyond question.

REFERENCES

Adams, G.A. (1986) Computer Technology: its impact on nursing practice. *Nursing Administration Quarterly*, **10**(2), 21–33.

Ashton, C. (1983) A computer system for drug prescribing and its impact on drug administration, in *Impact of Computers On Nursing* (eds M. Scholes *et al.*), Elsevier Science Publications BV, North Holland.

Ball, M.J. and Hannah, K.J. (1984) *Using Computers In Nursing*, Reston Publishing Company Inc., Reston, Virginia.

Beckmann, E. *et al.* (1981) Observation on computers in an intensive care unit. *Heart And Lung*, **10**(6), 1055–7.

Bell, P. and Catchpole, P. (1984) Management made easier. *Nursing Times*, **80**(36), 66–7.

Benton, D.C. (1988) An Evaluation Study Of CAL, in *Proceedings Of Second National Conference On The Use Of Computers In Health Care Education And Training*, NHS Training Authority, Sheffield.

Berrill, E.J. (1986) Electronic Nursing. *British Journal of Healthcare Computing*, **3**(2), 29–30.

Canter, D. (1984) Back to basics. *Nursing Times*, **80**(26), 49–50.

Catchpole, P. Avison, D. and Peart, S. (1987) The tale of two systems. *Nursing Times*, **83**(34), 57–8.

Clancy, W.J. (1979) Dialogue management for rule based tutorials. *International Journal of Computer Assisted Instruction*, **79**, 155–61.

Common Services Agency (1987) *Scottish Health Service Data Protection Act 1984 Subject Access Guidelines*, Common Services Agency, Edinburgh.

Cook, M. (1982) Using computers to enhance professional practice. *Nursing Times*, **78**(37), 1542–4.

Darley, K. (1983) All systems go. *Nursing Mirror*, **156**(4), 42–5.

Data Protection Registrar (1987) *Guideline 1 Data Protection Act 1984 Introduction to the Act*. (Revision 2) Plain English Campaign, (ed.), Harvest Printers Ltd, Macclesfield.

Department of Health and Social Security (1982) *First Report to the Secretary of State Steering Group On Health Services Information*, Her Majesty's Stationery Office, London.

Gebhardt, A.N. (1983) Developing a patient care program, in *Impact Of Computers On Nursing* (eds M. Scholes *et al.*) Elsevier Science Publications BV, North Holland.

Gerdin-Jelger, U. (1984) Nursing computers — the Swedish experience. *Nursing Times*, **80**(41), 44–5.

Grobe, S.J. (1984) Conquering computer cowardice. *Journal of Nurse Education*, **23**(6), 232–9.

Harrow, M. (1988) A computer for clinical nursing. *British Journal of Healthcare Computing*, **5**(1), 28–30.

Her Majesty's Stationery Office (1984) *Data Protection Act*, Her Majesty's Stationery Office, London.

Hoy, R. (1987) Unused potential. *Nursing Times*, **83**(34), 54.

Hunter, L. (1987) Keyboard rehabilitation. *Nursing Times*, **83**(32), 45–7.

Hyslop, A. and Jones, B. (1986) Putting AI into CAI. *British Computer Society Nursing Specialist News Letter*, **2**(2), 13–4.

McDonald, P. (1984) Writing a thesis on a word processor. *British Medical Journal*, **289**, 242–3.

McMenemin, J.M., Nadia, B.A., Hodsman, C., Murchie, J. and Kenny G.N.C. (1987) Applications of computers in clinical settings, in *Computers and their Application in Nursing* (ed. B. Koch and J. Rankin), Harper and Row, London.

Moores, B. and Murphy, A. (1984) Computerised duty rotas. *Nursing Times*, **80**(26), 47–8.

National Board for Nursing, Midwifery and Health Visiting for Scotland (1985) *Guidelines For Continuing Education Professional Studies 1 & 2*. National Board For Nursing, Midwifery and Health Visiting in Scotland, Edinburgh.

National Board for Nursing Midwifery and Health Visiting for Scotland (1987) *Report of the joint steering group on computer assisted learning*. National Board For Nursing, Midwifery and Health Visiting in Scotland, Edinburgh.

Norman, S.E. (1988) Users Perceptions Of CAL: An Evaluation, in *Proceedings Of Second National Conference on the Use of Computers in Health Care Education and Training*, NHS Training Authority, Sheffield.

Royal College Of Nursing (1984) *Report of the Working Group on Education and Training 1984 (Recommendations for Nursing Education through the Next Decade)*. Royal College of Nursing, London.

Royce, R. (1987) The reality Of implementing PAS. *British Journal Of Healthcare Computing*, **4**(6), 14 and 16.

Skinner, H.A. and Allen, B.A. (1983) Does the computer make a difference? computerised versus face to face self-report assessment of alcohol, drug and tobacco use. *Journal of Consulting and Clinical Psychology*, **51**(2), 267–75.

Smith, L.W. (1988) Microcomputer-based bibliographic searching. *Nursing Research*, **37**(2), 125–7.

Squire, P. (1982) Monitoring a sick pattern. *Nursing Mirror*, **154**(6), 20–2.

Stonier, T. (1988) Education and Training in the Age of Information, in *Proceedings Of Second National Conference on the Use of Computers in Health Care Education and Training*. NHS Training Aurthority, Sheffield.

Thomas, A. (1988) A strategy for NHS IT training. *British Journal of Healthcare Computing*, **5**(2), 17–8.

Townsend, I. and Norman, S. (1985) The Calgary Report. *Nurse Education Today*, **5**(4), 167–70.

United Kingdom Central Council for Nursing, Midwifery and Health Visiting (1987) *Project 2000 The Final Proposals Project Paper 9*, UKCC, London.

World Health Organization (1986) *Present and Potential Uses of Informatics and Telematics in Health*, WHO division of Information Support, ref: ISS/86/36, Geneva.

Chapter 12

Public speaking

DESMOND CORMACK

In this chapter 'public speaking' relates to the presentation of papers at conferences, study days, or seminars. The formality/informality of a presentation depends on the speaker, audience, purpose of the talk, and the venue. Much of this chapter applies equally to the large formal gathering and to the small informal gathering of colleagues. This type of speaking is similar in some ways to classroom teaching, or to the presentation of discussion papers within a classroom. Those two forms of 'public speaking' which are more aligned to teaching will not be discussed in this chapter, although some of the principles are obviously the same. Indeed, teaching can be a useful starting point from which to begin the development of public speaking skills. Certainly, opportunities for classroom speaking and/or the presentation of discussion papers can be used as a means of giving the confidence with which to speak to a larger and more formal audience, as can poster session presentation. See Sexton (1984) for a description of that specialist form of presentation.

Successful career development is undoubtedly dependent on an ability to be able to communicate (formally or informally) with large or small groups such as those attending study days and conferences.

CAN I SPEAK IN PUBLIC?

The short answer to this is 'Yes', if you want to. Indeed, virtually all registered nurses will probably have already done so. All of us have something important in our professional background to relate to others, but some may be reluctant to take on this responsibility in case they perform poorly. A fear of failure which is initially very strong in most of us, can be overcome by adequate preparation, starting with relatively easy speaking commitments, and by recognizing that speaking in public is a normal and natural ability, and is a responsibility of all members of all professions.

GETTING STARTED

A number of opportunities exist, both during and immediately after basic nurse training, which should be used to develop public speaking skills. Examples are the presentation of discussion papers in class, teaching practice with fellow students, contributing to the local in-service education programme, reading short papers at hospital study days, and collaborating in the presentation of a group paper at local conferences. Another possibility is for a group who wish to develop public speaking skills, to get together and create an in-service programme specifically designed to give participants the opportunity to give talks to the rest of the group for supportive and evaluative comment. Such a programme, led by a colleague with public speaking and/or teaching experience, can be an ideal way of getting started. All senior staff, particularly those with experience in public speaking have a clear responsibility to assist in the development of these skills in relatively junior and inexperienced staff. Indeed, many nursing conferences encourage and give the opportunity to nurses who will be speaking for the first time. With appropriate assistance, support and help from conference organizers and nursing colleagues generally, this approach can be used to enable major additions to be made to the pool of public speaking skills which are available in the profession.

The major reason for being invited to speak is the possession of a recognized expertise in relation to a specific subject area. This expertise may be rather general, the care of the elderly for example, or be rather more specialized and relate to topics such as nutrition and the elderly. Clearly, this expertise which you have must be made known to the profession generally in order that they can identify and locate you in order to extend an invitation to speak. An important means by which the profession can be informed of your expertise is for you to write and publish (see Chapter 14). Alternatively, you might respond to a 'Call for Abstracts' which is basically an open invitation from conference organizers to potential speakers to submit a summary/overview of a paper which they would like to present at the conference. The content of the 'Call for Abstracts' (see example below) will give a clear indication of the criteria upon which abstracts will be judged. Most commonly, but not exclusively, such requests for abstracts can be found in professional journals. On completion of an abstract for submission, ask a colleague to comment on your work and ensure that it complies with the requirements of the conference organizers.

Example Call for abstracts — 'The Application of Clinical Research', Dainbow General Hospital
(See accompanying advertisement for full conference details)

1. Abstracts are invited on all topics relevant to the theme of the conference from clinicians and researchers. In addition to research-

based papers, contributions are also invited from clinicians who wish to discuss the application of clinical research.

2. Each speaker will be allowed 30 minutes for the presentation, and 15 minutes for question/discussion.
3. All submitted abstracts will be considered by the conference planning committee, with decisions being made solely on the quality of the abstract. The closing date for submission of abstracts is . . . .
4. Abstracts should be submitted to . . . .

Format of Abstracts
Abstracts should be typed in double spacing on two separate sheets.
Sheet 1
   i. The title of the paper
  ii. Name and qualifications of the author
 iii. Work address
 iv. Details of present employment
   v. Audio-visual requirements
Sheet 2
 vi. Title of paper
vii. 300–400 word abstract

The abstract should include the aims and/or clinical application of a research study. It should also clearly demonstrate the application of research to clinical work.

Being invited to speak

Nurses who have a known expertise relating to the theme of the conference may be invited to give a talk without having to first go through the normal selection process by submitting an abstract. On receiving such an invitation there are a number of issues which require consideration before finally accepting or refusing it.

Can I speak on the subject? Although most conference organizers will have done their 'homework' prior to extending the invitation, it is not unknown for individuals to receive invitations to speak on subjects which are outside their area of expertise, or with which they are now out of touch. If you feel the invitation is outside your expertise, then immediately refuse it and give the reason. Clearly, invitations should never be accepted because a refusal would inconvenience the conference organizers, neither should they be accepted despite the subject being outside one's expertise, simply to give one experience in public speaking. The experienced *and* beginning speaker will be careful about which invitations to accept *and* which to refuse.

General content The invitation should include, in addition to the title, general guidelines about the content of the proposed talk. For example, if the title is 'The prevention of pressure sores', the conference organizers might indicate that you are being requested to speak about the prevention of pressure sores in the 1980s in relation to the elderly, in the UK and in relation to hospitalized patients. At this stage there may well be some room for negotiation in that the organizers will permit the exclusion and/inclusion of further related material which is more appropriate to your expertise. In any event, do not feel reluctant to 'negotiate' about the nature and content of an invited paper.

Where the talk will talk place   Details of the location of the conference are important and have implications for the ease with which you can travel there. Because the cost of travel can be considerable, as can the cost of one or two nights in a hotel, discuss whether or not conference organizers will cover travel and living costs. Not all conferences provide travel and/or living costs to those who present papers. In the event of these not being provided, your employer may consider sending you on the conference as a participant, and paying the appropriate costs in full or in part.

The date and time of conference   The date, time and duration of the conference will have implications for your own normal work commitments which may have to be postponed or done by others while you are away. Before formally accepting the invitation it is as well to make sure that time off work, or vacation/days off, can be used for travelling to and speaking at the conference.

Who will attend the conference?   An estimate of the size of the audience, a general account of the grades and background of the group who will attend, and whether or not non-nurses will attend needs to be known. This information will help you to decide whether or not you can prepare a paper to satisfy the needs of the particular audience.

Will the paper be published/circulated?   Conference papers are formally published by the organizers of some conferences, others are circulated to participants after the conference has ended. In either event you will wish to know of these arrangements well in advance in order that you can prepare your paper accordingly. Clearly, there will be considerable differences between a paper which is prepared for reading and subsequent publication, and one designed to provide 'general headings and notes' which you will use as an aide memoire for the presentation. Although most conference organizers tell speakers of this arrangement in advance, you can be 'caught out' by being asked to transfer rough notes into a publishable paper at short notice. If the papers are not to be published by the conference organizers, consider re-writing your talk for submission to a professional journal. Salome (1985) even suggests incorporating some question and answer material into the manuscript subsequently prepared for publication (see Chapter 14).

Accepting the invitation   Although an invitation may be made on an informal basis, over the telephone for example, it is subsequantly made in writing and includes details of the important aspects of the arrangements.

It is probably best to request a written invitation and to reply to it by letter, thus formalizing an arrangement which has previously been made personally and informally.

Preparing the talk

Having accepted the invitation to read the paper, work begins on preparing it. If you are a beginner, or if you have never talked in public before, preparation can be very time-consuming and might take up to two or three months of your spare time. Preparation begins by researching and reading around the subject in order to increase knowledge of it, and to become familiar with contemporary developments. Some papers will include a considerable amount of material which has been written by other people; a paper reviewing the current research into a subject area is an obvious example and should, of course, include detailed references and acknowledgements. If references are used in the talk, it is probably best to have these typed up and duplicated for distribution to all conference participants.

Place rough notes of key words and phrases on paper and subsequently arrange these into some form of logical sequence. These rough notes will form the basis of your paper, and will almost certainly go into several drafts before the final stage. Landsburg (1982) stressed that we must 'Organize, organize, organize' lecture notes.

As the final structure of the paper begins to emerge, decide how long it will be in terms of number of words. If you are placing every word of your talk on paper, a method used by some speakers, then establish how many words equate with a 30-minute talk for example. One way of doing this is to find a page of manuscript typed in double spacing and measure the amount of time you take to read it aloud. Reading a page of script to yourself (not aloud) requires far less time than it takes to read to an audience. If in doubt about the length of your paper then shorten it. An audience and chairman will forgive you for finishing slightly early. However, they are both likely, and entitled, to become restless and distracted if you exceed the agreed time. Also, it can be both embarrassing and stressful if the chairman suddenly tells you that 'Your 30 minutes is up and I regret that you now have to stop' or that 'You now have two minutes left in which to select and present material from the remaining pages of your paper'.

Important decisions

As the paper begins to develop there are a number of decisions which need to be made and which are important to the format, content and structure of the paper.

Discussions and questions may need to be accommodated at the end of the talk, although some speakers are quite happy for questions to be raised as an informal talk proceeds. The timing of questions is a matter for discussion between you and the person who will chair your session. In any event, make a decision, both in terms of when to allow questions and discussion, and the amount of time to be devoted to these.

Audiovisual aids can be used as a means of adding flavour and variety to a talk, in other instances they are a necessary and vital part of it. If you decide to use audiovisual aids, slides and overhead acetates for example, prepare these using expert advice from an audiovisual aids department, and fully test them in advance of the conference day, and check that facilities are available for their use. See Institution of Electrical Engineers (1974) and Essex-Lopresti (1979) for a discussion of how to prepare and use slides and overheads.

The format of notes vary depending on your experience and on whether you decide to present a formal speech or a rather more discursive dialogue with your audience. Full verbatim notes may be typed, in double spacing, on 6 × 4 in cards or on foolscap size paper. Whether cards or typing paper is being used the page/card number should be clearly placed on the front of each item in case the items become mixed up before or (worse still) during your presentation. Brewer (1988) was justifiably critical of the use of a full script (verbatim notes), suggesting that the main dangers were that the speaker could lose her place, or that the presentation could be dull and lifeless. Speakers are generally more informative and interesting if they use notes in the form of topics, headings, prompts and personal cues. Alternatively, you might place key words and/or phrases on the cards or sheets of paper. Many speakers, particularly on less formal occasions, use this form of brief notes in preference to a verbatim record of the entire talk.

On rare occasions an individual will deliver a talk with no notes whatsoever. These brave, or foolhardy, individuals are very rare and, in my experience, are usually either very good or very, very bad.

Notes contain additional prompts and pieces of information for personal use during the talk. The prompts might be written in red ink, appearing at the point in the talk where they will be used. Examples are:

- Present first slide here
- Check that everyone can read the slide
- Confirm that the people at the back can still hear me
- Check from my watch that I have reached the half-way stage
- Refer to handout No. 1
- Present second slide.

Writing the speech

Having generally prepared the structure and format of the speech, the full paper is now prepared. Because the content will vary from paper to paper, only the general principle relating to structure will be considered here.

Preliminary material

It is usual for speakers to be introduced by a chairman who either has responsibility for chairing the entire conference, part of it, or an individual presentation. In either event the role of the chairman will be to introduce you and, having previously obtained some personal details about your professional experiences and background, sets the scene for your particular presentation. An example of how your paper might look, in terms of structure is:

Thanking the chairman who has introduced you is a useful start and helps to 'break the ice'. Thanking him/her for the introduction and/or the invitation to speak at the conference is normal practice.

Personal details, in addition to those provided by the chairman, may be provided by you. For example, if the chairman has not mentioned that you were previously employed as a community psychiatric nurse, and this aspect of your background is relevant to the audience, feel free to inform them. This time is used to form a relationship with the audience and might include such informal social comments as the pleasure which you have in visiting this particular institution or city.

Administrative details of your presentation might be discussed here. For example, you might remind the audience that there will be a 30-minute talk followed by 15-minute discussion period. Alternatively, you might invite questions during your talk. If handouts are to be used, and they have been distributed to members of the audience on entry to the hall, ensure that everyone has a copy before starting.

The title and purpose of the talk is then repeated, even although this has already been done by the chairman, followed by a statement of its general aim. This might be followed by a brief overview of the entire paper, an overview which outlines its parts. For example, you might say: 'In the first part of this paper I will present an overview of the major components of the nursing process. Secondly, I will discuss each part of the nursing process in detail, and describe its use in my particular hospital. Finally, I will discuss the advantages and disadvantages of moving to the use of the nursing process'. The purpose of this introduction is to prepare the audience for what they are about to hear. This preparation will help them to assimilate and remember the material which is to follow.

The body of the talk comes next and will constitute the major part in terms of time. This material, as with the rest of the talk, is presented in a logical, coherent and unhurried fashion. In writing the speech, full use should be made of major headings, sub-headings and sub-sub-headings. Although the audience do not see the headings, they can be used by you to indicate when new topics are being moved on to, or where a sub-topic is in fact part of a major topic. Below headings, you may wish to make a statement such as 'Now I will move on to consider the position of student nurses'.

The concluding statement will draw the paper to a close and is used to remind the audience of the major topics covered in your paper. For example, you may say; 'In summary, this paper has dealt with the following topics...' This will allow the audience to expect your contribution to end soon, and to anticipate a final concluding statement such as 'Thank you very much for giving me this opportunity to meet with you to discuss...' and to give them a cue for the customary applause.

At the conference

Preparations for your contribution continue on arrival at the conference venue, your personal arrangements being in addition to the more general ones which have been made by your hosts.

Visit the hall or room in which you will read your paper and 'get the feel' of the physical surroundings in which you will present it.

Audiovisual aids, including the microphone, are tested and adapted to suit your particular needs. If a microphone is not to be used then ask someone to stand at the back of the room and indicate whether or not they can hear you when using a particular level of voice. If audiovisual aids such as a slide or overhead projector are being used, establish who will operate the machinery, who will adjust the lights if that will be required, who will operate the screens and curtains and who (if anyone) will be available to offer assistance if the audiovisual machinery breaks down.

Prepare the stage props by examining and, if necessary, altering the position of the table, chair, microphone and lectern. Be sure that, within reasonable limits, the stage and its props are suitable to you. The height of the lectern should be tested, if there is no such facility then consider where you will place your notes when speaking. It is probably as well to request that a jug of water and a glass be made available to you. Although you may not particularly wish to drink the water, this can be a useful means of obtaining a few seconds 'thinking time' when considering a reply to a question for example.

Presenting the paper

The period immediately prior to presentation, when waiting and listening to the chairman's introduction for example, frequently results in a little nervousness. This is quite normal, and something which almost all speakers experience. Your carefully prepared notes will guide you through the talk, and your inserted cues and prompts will provide additional information for your use. At the beginning of a presentation some inexperienced speakers are tempted to begin with a 'quick apology' for their inexperience. Such an apology is always unnecessary and deflects from the quality of your personal contribution. You are there because you are an expert on the subject, and your inexperience as a speaker is quite understandable. Nervousness is something which you will be much more aware of than will be the audience.

Although your notes will tell you what to say and will include some prompts such as 'pause' or an emphasized word being in BLOCK CAPITALS, your notes will not tell you how to project your material. Changes in tone, emphasis, variation in speed, body language and eye contact with individual members of the audience are things which will be learned by experience. However, there are some techniques (such as inserting comments and cues in your notes) which will help. These include:

- Writing your notes in a way which highlights key words, underlining points to be emphasized, using capital letters and spaces for dramatic effect, giving instructions such as 'pause' will generally guide you on how to present the material. Such an example is:
  The view of my colleagues is that we will not compromise on standards of patient care. I invite you to reflect on the result of compromise. (PAUSE) I submit that we must never deviate from our goal to make high quality care available to all patients.

With experience, you will develop the ability to accommodate any spontaneous response, such as applause, from the audience. Additionally, you will learn how and when to inject short or long pauses in order to let a particular point 'sink in'. Do not hesitate to use body language to improve communication with the audience. Virtually all experienced speakers make full use of a variety of non-verbal communication techniques, an important example is 'achieving a presence' by standing erect when talking. Alternatively, when meeting with a small and informal group, a speaker might maximize participants' contribution to discussion by sitting with them, or by standing among or near to participants.

Your thorough knowledge of the subject of your speech will add to confidence and skill in presentation. Indeed, this confidence will eventually enable you to make less use of your notes, or to deviate from them slightly when appropriate.

The time spent in planning the content and structure of notes will result in a fluent presentation. Previous practice at reading and timing the material either alone, to a friend or into a tape recorder will also help greatly. These 'practice runs' will result in a conversational style of presentation rather than a reading/dictation style.

When you are finished, make sure the audience know it. This might be done by using a phrase such as 'Thank you very much for your time and the invitation to present this paper'.

Your previous arrangement with the chairman will determine the way in which you handle 'question time'. He/she may invite questions and generally 'chair' the question time. Alternatively, the arrangement made may be that questions are directed straight to you. Some questions can be rather vague, complex, unpredictable, and sometimes meaningless. Particularly for beginners, questions are best handled through the chair, enabling the chairperson to help and support the speaker. However, bear in mind that you are there because you are the expert on the subject and almost certainly know more about it than most others at the conference. A few hints in relation to questions may be of value:

- Always accept the questioner's point of view, although you may disagree with it
- Clarify questions which are vague
- Admit to not knowing the answer to any specific question
- Redirect questions to the audience if you feel that they may have an answer you do not have
- Avoid getting involved in a long debate with one individual in the audience
- Accept your limitations (remember, nobody knows everything about anything).

Finally, enjoy the give and take of question and discussion time as an important learning experience. Public speaking and discussion is as much a learning experience for the speaker as for the audience.

CONCLUSION

There is no doubt that the development of public speaking skills, in the broadest meaning of the term, will greatly enhance career development both in terms of what a nurse can give to and get from professional nursing. This applies to all professional nurses whether they be clinicians, researchers, administrators or teachers, and whether or not they are, or will be seeking promotion.

Regard public speaking as being a responsibility of every professional. Indeed, given that the term has an extremely broad definition in this chapter, it is probable that virtually all readers will already have had some experience, and that this is reflected in curriculum vitae content.

REFERENCES

Brewer, S. (1988) How to speak effectively. *Nursing Standard*, **2**(38), 19.
Essex-Lopresti, M. (1979) How to: Use an overhead projector. *Medical Teacher*, **1**(1), 9–15.
Institution of Electrical Engineers (1974) *Handbook for Speakers*. The Institution of Electrical Engineers, London.
Landsburg, D. (1982) Nine clues to effective presentation. *Supervisory Management*, **27**(4), 28–33.

Salome, P. (1985) Double-duty speeches can help you publish! *Nursing Success Today*, **2**(3), 9–10.
Sexton, D. (1984) Presentation of research findings: The poster session. *Nursing Research*, **33**(6), 374–5.

Chapter 13

Conference attendance

DESMOND CORMACK

Although this chapter title refers only to 'conference' attendance, the term should be regarded as also referring to attending study days, seminars and other similar events. It also refers to 'workshops', a specialized form of conference which Stevens (1977) described as a concentrated group educational experience with its own unique characteristics. That writer gave an excellent account of how to organize and participate in a successful workshop.

Conferences vary in length, ranging from the locally organized one-day conference, the two- or three-day national event, longer ones of up to one week in duration, and the increasing number of international events relating to health care generally or nursing in particular. The considerable provision of nursing conferences presents much opportunity for making use of them in relation to your career development. As with other aspects of professional development, attendance at appropriate conferences is a normal and natural component, rather than an optional extra. In recent years the variety and range of conference topics has enlarged many fold, with a large number of nurses having gained the ability and experience to contribute to, and participate in, this form of professional information exchange. The internationalization of nursing, accompanied with the recognition of the need for fuller and more rapid information exchange has resulted in a considerable growth in the number of conferences which are addressed by international nursing figures. Similarly, it is now common practice for local, regional and national specialist groups to organize regular activities of these types.

PURPOSE OF CONFERENCES

The most obvious purpose of any conference is to give participants the opportunity to listen to the delivery of papers by experts in a particular field. More importantly, attendance provides an opportunity to enter into discussion and debate with regard to the issues raised. The questions generated during formal and informal discussion periods gives opportunity to challenge the views of 'experts' and requires speakers to explain and defend their points of view. Indeed, the formal presentation of papers is only one (although important) part of the conference. Thus, the inter-action between speaker and participants contributes considerably to the value of any conference. Without this speaker–participant dialogue, the organizers might just as well have arranged for speakers to send a copy of each talk to every participant. Another crucial element in attendance is the opportunity for meeting with colleagues and continuing the discussions of presented papers. This view was shared by McKenzie (1986) who wrote: '...one of the main attractions of a conference is the opportunity to meet with others working in the same area as oneself.'

Such opportunities are made much more possible if the conference is a residential one. Indeed, one of the factors in influencing your de-cision to attend may be whether or not the conference is residential. Al-though invariably more expensive than a non-residential conference, the increased opportunity to meet colleagues usually makes the additional cost well worthwhile (see also Chapter 20).

Conference types

A number of types of conference structure exist, clearly influencing deci-sions as to whether or not you attend. For example, it may be 'topic related' and be concerned with such issues as incontinence, aggression, disorienta-tion, cross-infection, immobility or anxiety. The intended audience at such events will be individuals whose work has these subjects as a particular focus. Others might be specialty related and cover broader issues such as community nursing, the care of the elderly, theatre nursing, paediatric nursing or intensive care work. These have a broader base and are de-signed to attract participants from these particular specialties. Broad issues are the subject of some conferences which deal with topics which are of relevance to nurses from all specialities. Examples of this type are meetings which address such issues as ethics related to nursing, nursing politics, nursing research and the use of information technology. Another type is that which is role related, and is primarily directed at those who are working in administration, teaching or research. Another is that which is directed at a specific level of staff such as staff nurses, charge nurses, nursing officers or senior nursing administrators. Finally, an increasing number of conferences are multidisciplinary and focus on issues which are of common interest to physicians, nurses, social workers, psychologists, and other members of the health care team.

Conference advertising

Conference advertising is done by a range of means from local (in-house) notices to those adverts which appear in the national and international journals. Prior notice of those which are primarily local in nature will usually appear in publications such as hospital newsletters, or on the local notice board. Alternatively, you might hear of a local conference from a colleague who works in another locality. Although such conferences are primarily for staff of that area, admission might be obtained via contacts in these localities.

Information regarding national and international conferences is usually obtained from two major sources. First, from professional bodies who organize them, the Royal College of Nursing for example. It is usual, however, for this information to be made known initially to the memberships of these organizations. It is also usual for their members to be given preferential treatment in terms of the cost of attending, and possibly in relation to obtaining a place if it is oversubscribed. Second, the national and international nursing press carry advertisements for a full range of conferences. Those journals which are generalist in nature, for example, the *Nursing Times*, carry notices relating to all kinds of conferences irrespective of their nursing specialty. Others, such as the *Journal of Gerontological Nursing*, carry advertisements in relation to that particular specialty. Thus, it is necessary to keep up to date with the materials contained both in specialist and generalist journals. Also read non-nursing journals such as the *British Medical Journal* in order to locate conferences which are primarily medically oriented, or those which have a multidisciplinary focus.

Should I attend?

The answer to this question is made following a full examination of the nature and scope of the conference, and its relationship to present career and future career development. Although some advertisements carry sufficient information upon which to judge the relevance of the conference, others carry a limited amount of detail. If the information is insufficient, contact the organizers and obtain a full breakdown of the speakers, subjects covered and possible range of backgrounds of participants.

Usually, detailed information about the conference accurately reflects its title. On other occasions, you may find that the content of the conference material is only partially reflected in its title. A decision can therefore only be made by obtaining full information.

The cost of conference attendance is another crucial issue. Invariably, the greater the distance between the conference and your place of work, the greater the cost. Additionally, longer conferences are proportionately cheaper per day of attendance than are shorter ones. Overseas conferences are even more expensive and are rightly regarded as the kind of thing that might be done only a small number of times in a professional lifetime. In summary, the question 'Should I attend?' can only be answered when you have closely examined the relevance of the conference material to your present and future career development, the cost of the conference, the amount of time that will require to be devoted to travelling to and attending it, and the availability of time and financial resources.

Planning conference attendance

Initially, obtain full information regarding the purpose and scope of the conference, and make a judgement as to whether or not it coincides with the needs of your career development. Next, consider the financial and time resources which are required for attendance. Given that it is normal for employers to support the professional development of staff, it may be that you will be seeking financial and other forms of support from your employer.

Because very few (if any) employers have unlimited resources to invest in staff development they tend to prioritize the many requests for the support which they receive. Attention needs to be given to an application for support for conference attendance, as does the extent to which you are, or are not, willing to contribute financially or otherwise to the overall cost of attendance.

Reason for conference attendance

When applying for financial support and/time off to attend a conference, include a copy of the conference programme, supported by a clear and concise explanation of the reasons for wishing to attend. Prior to formulating a formal request for support, discuss it with the appropriate person in your organization. Ideally, obtain an 'in principle' agreement before formally submitting the request. The request letter should also contain a clear indication of the reasons for wishing to attend the conference, along with details of the costs and other forms of support which are being requested.

Attending the conference

Although the major purpose of attending a conference is to listen to, and learn from, the speakers there are a number of additional aspects which should be borne in mind. Prior to the conference, 'read around' the subject in order to update yourself. This activity is particularly useful as a preparation for contributing to the discussion following the presentation of papers, and to information discussion with other participants in the 'free time'.

Note taking

During the presentation of papers it is essential that notes be taken with regard to the content. Ideally, these are fully written up or placed on a recording machine as soon as possible after the presentation. One of the advantages of residential courses is that part of the free time in the evening can be used for this purpose. The notes can also be used for reference during the subsequent discussion and/or in the formulation of questions as the end of the presentation.

At some conferences, particularly the larger national or international ones, participants have to make a choice (often in advance of the conference dates) with regard to which of the concurrent sessions to attend. Occasionally, a choice will have to be made with regard to attending one presentation out of three or more which are being made at one time. Making this choice can be difficult if more than one of the papers on offer is of particular interest. This problem can be overcome by either obtaining the notes taken by a colleague who has attended another presentation, or by asking someone to obtain an extra copy of handouts or other material made available at those which you are unable to attend.

Asking questions

It is usual for participants to be given the opportunity to ask questions or raise points for discussion at the end of each presentation or session. Because the amount of time for questions/points for discussion is invariably limited, it is probable that a relatively small number of participants will be able to take advantage of this opportunity. In fairness to the speaker, and to other participants, questions should be short and to the point. Nothing is more frustrating than to find that a 'question' from the floor is in fact a protracted and complicated 'mini-lecture' on the subject. Prior to asking a question or raising a point for discussion, make a written note of it, then read it to the speaker. An example of such a question might be: 'You have mentioned two similar methods of dealing with incontinence in the elderly. From your experience of using these two systems, do you have any preference?'

Although not all participants will have the opportunity to raise question/ points for discussion, it is as well to formulate a question in the course of the presentation, or during subsequent question time. If you have no opportunity to ask the question at this point, there may well be a chance to raise it with the speaker or with other participants in subsequent informal discussions.

Informal discussions

All conferences, whether resident or non-resident, allow some time for informal discussion over coffee, during meal times and in the 'free time' in the evenings. This time is used for informal discussions with speakers and other participants. Because many conference presentations are relatively short, with some offering little subsequent opportunity for questions, the issues raised by speakers can and should be more fully discussed with them and other participants. These reciprocal exchanges of views are important learning experiences for the 'expert' speakers and participants alike.

Networking

By their nature, conferences draw together a group of people with similar interests and, frequently, with similar backgrounds. Opportunities are taken to establish informal and long-term links with colleagues, such contacts being of mutual advantage. Some conferences provide a list of the names and contact addresses of all participants, this can be used to identify the individuals with whom you wish to explore the possibility of continued contact. If no such list is available, it falls on you to identify and make contact with others who can form part of a professional network system (see also Chapter 20).

Conference documents

The amount of documents provided prior to, and during, conferences varies considerably. Some provide only a programme which is lacking in detail. Others provide a more detailed programme, a list of participants and a range of 'handouts' produced by individual speakers. If these handouts include a summary of individual papers, they are of particular importance. I suggest that all conference papers, particularly those relating to individual presentations, be carefully collected and filed. They will be of special value when writing up a report of the conference, and in developing and continuing contact with the speakers and other participants.

Exhibitions

Many conferences, particularly the national and international ones, include exhibitions of equipment and/or books relating to the subject of the conference. These are clearly a useful adjunct to the presentation and discussion of papers.

Associated visits

Some conferences offer professional visits to clinical and associated facilities in the vicinity. The numbers of places on such visits are frequently limited and may have to be booked at the same time as the conference application is made. Frequently these are offered on a 'first come, first served' basis, underlining the need for application to be made as early as possible.

ADVANTAGES OF CONFERENCES

Usually, conferences provide the participants with up-to-date material which has not yet been published or which reflect the speakers' views which have been more fully developed since publication. However, unfortunately, some speakers may present material which has been previously published, or which has not been up-dated since publication or since a previous conference presentation.

Conference attendance offers an opportunity for informal discussion and further exploration of its subject matter. The importance of renewing old professional contacts, making new ones, and of networking generally cannot be overemphasized. They also enable you to regenerate and maintain professional enthusiasm.

DISADVANTAGES OF CONFERENCES

Conference attendance can be costly in terms of finance and the time involved. For this reason, make sure that the subject matter is relevant to present and future professional functioning. Because of the costs, both in time and money, a relatively small number of nurses can attend, highlighting the need to give full and detailed feedback to colleagues who are unable to attend.

The quality of conference presentations can range from the poor to the excellent, although it is unusual for an entire conference to be of poor quality. Additionally, the level of the presented material may, or may not, meet your specific requirements. It is usually possible to make a judgement as to whether the quality and/or level of the presented materials will meet your needs by reference to the conference publicity documents. In particular, carefully examine the qualifications and backgrounds of the speakers, the objectives of the conference and the audience to which it is directed.

CONFERENCE EVALUATION

Conferences can, and should, be evaluated from a number of perspectives which are of considerable interest to you, your employer and/or other sponsor, colleagues who are unable to attend, and to those who arranged the conference and contributed to it. Some conference organizers will invite participants to complete an evaluation form and return it to them anonymously. Whether or not such a request is made, consider evaluating the conference using the following criteria:

1. Was it of value in terms of its cost and duration?
2. Were the preliminary papers sufficiently detailed to give a clear indication of quality, level and subject matter?
3. Was the structure, level and general quality of the material adequate? How did the presented material relate to that contained in the conference publicity?

4. Was the quality, experience and professional knowledge of the speakers appropriate to the level of the conference? In general, was the presentation of speakers adequate?
5. Did the speakers make appropriate use of audiovisual teaching aids?
6. Were participants fully encouraged to provide items for question and/or discussion?
7. Did the conference organization provide reasonable time for making informal contact with other participants?
8. Are the proceedings to be published in full (free or at a cost)? Alternatively, did individual speakers provide abstracts of their talks and/or other handouts?
9. Were associated exhibitions and/or professional visits organized as part of the conference?
10. What was the quality of the general administrative and domestic arrangements, including those relating to the provision of accommodation, if the conference was a residential one?
11. Finally, would you recommend that a further similar conference be attended by a colleague with similar professional interests and background to your own?

AFTER THE CONFERENCE

The major function of conference attendance is to influence your professional development in terms of knowledge and/or skills development with a view to optimizing your level of functioning as a nurse clinician, manager, teacher or research. Although benefits may not necessarily be evident in the short term, there is little doubt that attendance at appropriate professional conferences will positively influence your performance in the medium and long term.

Another function of attendance is to enable you to inform and educate those colleagues who were unable to attend. This can and should be done in one or more ways. For example, you might 'write up' a paper and circulate it to colleagues. One way of 'getting the feel' of how such a paper might be structured is to read one which has been successfully submitted for publication. For example see Houston (1987) and Walker (1988). Alternatively, you might give a talk on the conference content, followed by a discussion of selected issues. The need to share conference information was emphasized by Brewin-Wilson (1985) who concluded that the best way of maximizing the value of conferences was for attenders to 'share the fruits of the meetings they attend with their colleagues who stay at home'. Indeed, it may be argued that the selection of those who will be given employers' support to attend should be strongly influenced by the ability and willingness of the applicant to 'report back'.

REFERENCES

Brewin-Wilson, D. (1985) Getting maximum mileage from your next nursing conference. *R.N.*, **48**(4), 43–5.

Houston, M. (1987) Conference report: research and the midwife. *Midwifery* **4**(2), 91–2.

McKenzie, G. (1986) Editorial: Do conferences serve a useful function? *Nurse Education Today*, **6**, 47.

Stevens, B. (1977) The successful workshop: How to bring it off!! *Nurse Educator*, **2**(1), 16–20.

Walker, J. (1988) Editorial: Pathways for progress in nurse education. *Nurse Education Today*, **8**, 249–50.

Chapter 14

Writing for professional publication

DESMOND CORMACK

One of the hallmarks of a profession is that it produces and records a body of knowledge which is specific to that particular profession. Invariably, this knowledge is contained in the form of written material. In order for that material to be generally available to the profession, it is necessary for it to be published. Although a small amount of such written information remains unpublished, for example in the form of some higher degree theses, it requires to be made widely available via publication. Thus, the primary reason for the publication of materials by nurses is to maintain the existence of nursing as a profession. Styles (1978) expresses it thus: 'The primary reason to publish is because the future of the profession depends upon it. . . . Not to publish is an aching nothingness in a part of one's professional soul.'

This general view of the necessity for nurses to publish reflects the requirement that it is the responsibility of all individuals and groups of nurses irrespective of their area or level of functioning. It is a professional requirement of clinicians, administrators, teachers and researchers.

During recent years the impetus for regarding writing for publication as involving all nurses has gained momentum. Initially, much of the published material generated by the profession was produced by a relatively small number of its members. These publications were primarily produced by nurse teachers, nurse researchers and nurse managers. The current position has now dramatically changed in that a large volume of published material has been written by nurse clinicians.

Nurses are fortunate in that the development of writing skills forms a central part of initial training. In particular, the production of essays, extended pieces of course-work, clinical and research projects has produced a profession with a high competence level in producing written work. In many instances nurse training schools are assisting students to further develop these writing skills to enable them to take the relatively small step towards producing work for publication. Brosnan and Kovalesky (1980) suggested that all nursing education programmes should include some instruction on how to write for publication. They suggested that nurse teachers might give students the option of producing written assignments in publication format, rather than in the usual essay or care-plan format. Under the guidance of someone who is experienced in writing for publication, students can easily be taught to adapt their normal (frequently clinically oriented) writing style to produce a paper for submission to a journal. Wooley and Hatcher (1986) described how they taught their nursing students to 'shape' their major written assignments for publication, and instructed them on the construction of a query letter to a potential journal publisher.

In addition to contributing to the development of the nursing profession, writing for publication has other more personal motivations. White (1987) surveyed 226 nurses who had published an article during the previous one-year period. One of the questions in that survey sought to determine why authors published these particular manuscripts. Fifty-two respondents indicated that they had written the article because the subject was of interest to self and others; 44 wished to contribute to nursing theory; 25 used the article as a means of reporting research findings; 24 wrote the manuscript because 'the idea was novel'; 11 writers had been encouraged to do so by colleagues, and 37 indicated that the manuscripts were solicited by the journals. Interestingly, only 7 respondents indicated career advancement as being a reason for writing the paper. Although the 'publish or perish' ethic is not presently considered to be fundamental to success in nursing, there is much evidence to suggest that it is becoming increasingly so. See Cormack (1984) for a full discussion of writing for publication.

APPROACHES TO WRITING FOR PUBLICATION

A variety of approaches are used in writing for publication, these depending on the purpose of the publication and the type of material which is to be presented. Needless to say, it is necessary to decide on the type of approach to be used prior to writing the manuscript. The following are examples of the type of approaches that might be used.

The manuscript might be used to:

- Speculate and raise issues in nursing generally, or in relation to a specific specialty. Implicit in the development of any profession is the need to challenge existing views and to speculate about the future. As the nursing profession develops, new issues are generated and become the subject of wide debate before conclusions are reached.
- Influence opinion by presenting arguments for/or against a particular aspect of nursing practice, education, research or management. Each individual nurse has an important contribution to make to the develop-

ment of the general opinion of the nursing profession as it relates to internal and wider considerations.

- Clarify ideas which have not yet been fully developed on a personal or wider basis, and which require discussion with others.
- Inform others of new approaches to nursing care which one has developed personally, or in association with others. Such an exchange of information enables others to avoid 're-inventing the wheel'. This type of article might focus on case studies, or deal with the general aspects of nursing practice, administration, teaching or research.
- Review the literature relating to a specific aspect of nursing. In addition to informing the reader of the literature on a topic, such an article will include a critical analysis of the published materials.
- Report research findings, usually in the form of a description of part of a research project, or a summary of the entire study.
- Examine historical developments in nursing by describing how current practice has been influenced by historical events, and speculating about how these might influence the future.
- Contribute to nursing theory by presenting a philosophical form of discussion which will enable an understanding of current nursing practice, and provide directions for future progress.
- Finally, publishing can be used as a means of 're-packaging' existing knowledge in a way which will improve understanding of the material, or which applies existing knowledge to novel situations.

WRITING OPPORTUNITIES

Writing for publication is not confined to the preparation of journal articles. Other opportunities include writing or editing textbooks, contributing chapters to textbooks, writing book reviews, letters to the professional journals, and contributions to the non-nursing professional press and to the general (non-health care) press. Many of the references contained in the Further Reading list reflect the variety of writing opportunities for nurses.

For the purpose of illustration the remainder of this chapter will focus on the preparation of an article for publication. This decision is justified on two grounds: first, it is the type of professional publication with which all nurses are familiar. Second, publication in the form of journal articles is the type of publishing opportunity which is readily available.

WRITING A JOURNAL ARTICLE

The following is an outline of the stages of preparing and submitting an article for publication. At first sight, this process may appear to be rather long and complicated. However, it is a relatively simple and 'mechanical' activity with the stages representing nothing more than a series of ground rules.

Previous experience

The basis for preparing a manuscript is the pre-existing clinical, administrative, teaching or research experience (or combinations of these). Inherent in these experiences, and in initial nurse training, is the ability to write for a variety of other purposes. Thus, the starting point for any professional nurse is a combination of previous experience and existing writing skills.

Generation of idea

Reflection on previous nursing experience, and on your current area of functioning, will produce ideas for a publication topic. These ideas are produced by asking questions such as 'What am I doing that others might be interested in learning about; which areas of nursing are poorly understood and in need of discussion; in which areas is there a conflict between nursing knowledge and practice; are there accepted areas within nursing with which I am in strong disagreement; which new issues are currently being discussed and about which there requires to be more speculation; and which areas of nursing require to be the subject of greater research?'

Reading around the subject

Once a general idea has been identified, the next step is to read published materials on the subject in order to learn about the subject, and to determine the extent to which it has, or has not, been addressed in the literature. Additionally, this activity can be used to identify those journals which deal with this particular subject area and to learn about successful article construction.

Refining the idea

Personal experience, combined with a review of the literature, will enable the general subject area to be further refined. It is not unusual to begin with a general topic such as 'psychiatric nursing in the community' and, as a result of reading the literature on the subject, begin to realize that a more relevant and specific focus might be 'the care of the demented elderly in the community' for example. At this stage, or possibly earlier, it will be useful to discuss the topic of the potential publication with a colleague or some other person who is familiar with writing for publication and/or with the subject matter.

Identify target readership

Identifying a possible target readership is necessary from two points of view. First, in order to select an appropriate journal(s) and to ensure that the article is written with a specific readership in mind. Some articles deal with subjects which are of general interest; one relating to continuing education for example. Others are much more specific, the prevention of cross-infection in surgical wards is such an example. Similarly, some journals have a general content and readership, the *American Journal of Nursing* and the *Nursing Times* are such examples. Other journals are much more specific, they include the *Journal of Gerontological Nursing* and *Nurse Education Today*. At this stage, the writer is beginning to 'match up' the article with a specific type of readership and, by definition, professional nursing journal.

Article outline

Writers use a variety of techniques for 'getting started' when beginning work on an article. One approach is to write down a series of general headings and/or ideas which will become the focus of the paper. These items, each of which might be one, two or three words long, need not necessarily be written in the correct sequence at this stage. The next task is to rearrange these items in an appropriate order which will constitute the three major parts of the paper, that is the beginning/introduction, the body of the paper, and then the conclusion. This series of headings, which may run into no more than a single page, is then extended by developing each of its parts into a few lines. The resultant two to three page general outline will form the skeleton of the paper from which the full article will develop.

Selecting possible journals

The previous literature review, and a familiarity with the better known nursing publications, will enable a small number of relevant journals to be identified. A good nursing library will contain a selection of journals, enabling decisions regarding which are most appropriate for the article. Another good source of possible journals is the numerous reference texts which deal with nursing indexes, research abstracts and bibliographies. Swanson and McCloskey (1986) provide some details of publishing policies and practices of 139 journals, all of which publish articles written by, and relating to, nurses.

Professional nursing, and the literature which it produces is becoming more internationalized. When writing an article for publication, it is desirable that you consider publishing in countries other than your own.

Sending a query letter

Swanson and McCloskey (1986) reported that the majority of journal editors welcomed receipt of a query letter in advance of manuscript submission. Although it is generally accepted that manuscripts are sent to only one journal at a time, a query letter containing an outline of the manuscript can be sent to a number of journals simultaneously. Such a letter will contain an overview of the proposed article (a single page summary for example), and indicate how the material will be of interest to the journal's readership. Additionally, it will inform the editor of your credentials, qualifications and present work position. Vivas (1982) suggests that it is generally considered advisable to send a query letter to a journal outlining a proposed article before sending in the manuscript. In addition to making contact with the editor, you are able to minimize the possibility of rejection at a later stage. The reply to the query letter may well contain guidance as to the emphasis and/or particular focus which will maximize the possibility of acceptance. The name and address of the editor, to whom the query letter should be addressed, will usually be found on the title page of the journal.

Refereed journals are those which use a panel of independent 'experts' to read and evaluate submitted manuscripts. Swanson and McCloskey (1986) reported that in their survey of 139 journal editors over 87% defined their journals as refereed publications. Typically, these editors reported that received manuscripts were distributed to experts selected from an established group of reviewers. Decisions on the manuscript were then based on the reports of reviewers, with subsequent mediation by the editor. Clayton and Boyle (1981) provide an excellent insight into the notion of referees/non-refereed journal publication.

Selecting a journal

At this stage, begin to focus on one specific journal for which the manuscript will be prepared and subsequently submitted. A combination of the already prepared framework, the journal guide for contributors, and the reply(ies) to a query letter (if one was sent) will help you to make decisions about the format and content of the finished manuscript. At this stage you are writing for a specific audience in a specific journal and working within the constraints and guidelines of one particular publication. A 'Guide for Contributors' is normally found inside each, or most, issues of a journal. If not, it can be obtained on request from the journal editor.

WRITING THE MANUSCRIPT

It is quite normal to write two or more drafts before reaching the final manuscript. The previously prepared framework is used to provide the structure of the article, with each of the framework parts being elaborated on and developed to achieve the required amount of detail and length. One way of achieving this is to double the length of the framework to achieve a first draft, increase the detail and discussion to again double the length of the manuscript, then write a final draft which approximates the final desired length. A writer who is familiar with the subject matter will be able to write as little or as much on a particular topic as is necessary to conform to the requirements of a particular journal. At this stage, decisions are made regarding the material which is to be included/excluded from the manuscript. Similarly, attention is paid to the language used and to writing style. Thus, you consider content, structure and style.

Content

The manuscript will contain and relate to a major central idea or statement which is clearly expressed and made known to the reader. In addition to containing some reference to previously published material on the subject, the paper will contain sufficient additional supporting material to convince the reader that the paper is well considered and of importance. A balance is struck between stating the obvious, and making assumptions regarding the prior knowledge of the reader. As the manuscript develops, it should be read by colleagues of the kind who will become the eventual readership, with a view to ensuring that the material is clear and meaningful, and that it fully addresses the major topic which is embodied in the article title.

Structure

The general structure of the manuscript will be the introduction, the body of the paper, and finally the conclusion and/or summary. The introduction is used to set the scene for the remainder of the paper, and to provide sufficient background information to enable the reader to make meaning of the content. It is usual to make reference to other published material on the subject in the introductory part of the manuscript. The body of the paper contains a full discussion of the subject matter and, because of its relative length, invariably contains a number of sub-parts. The concluding section summarizes the preceding material and is used to state the relevance of the paper and indicate how the material contributes to knowledge relating to nursing practice, administration, research or education.

The use of headings and sub-headings will enable the reader to identify the major parts and sub-parts of the article, and will enable (and interlink) the movement from one part of the subject matter to another. Examination of published articles will give a clear indication of how and why headings and sub-headings are used in these respects.

Within the introduction, body and conclusion an attempt is made to present the material in a clear order which may be chronological or of some other type of sequence. Thus, the 'flow' of the paper, and the order in which its parts appear, is intended to assist the readers' understanding of the material.

Just as the flow of the material is assisted by attention to the major and minor parts of the paper, each of the paragraphs and sentences are written in a specifically determined sequence which adds to the 'readability' of the manuscript.

During the initial phase of writing a manuscript, it is not unusual for writers to have a number of relatively disjointed ideas which are written in a seemingly random sequence. As the paper progresses, these ideas and statements are continuously arranged and rearranged in order to ensure the production of a paper which has a meaningful and logical sequence. By writing in pencil and/or on one side of a page of paper it becomes easier to 'cut and paste' parts of the paper in order to rearrange them.

Style

Although poor writing style is the least frequent reason for rejection of a manuscript, the expressed ideas and content being more important, attention to writing style can improve the possibility of success. The language used in the paper must be appropriate to the intended readership. In addition to using professional experience to achieve and make use of an appropriate form of words, examine published manuscripts in the journal of choice in order to get some feel for the general style which is used.

All sentences and individual words are closely examined in order to ensure that their meaning is unambiguous. A critical review of the manuscript by a colleague should give some indication of the clarity of the work. The following guidelines may be of value in relation to achieving effective writing style.

Develop a *personal* writing style, rather than attempting to 'copy' that which has been developed by other writers. Each individual constructs a highly individualized writing style which operates within the framework of a generally accepted structure. Thus, although the structure of your paper may be similar to that of others, the style will be relatively individualized.

Effective writing style and the development of structure is helped by reading the professional literature. An article which is published represents a 'success' in that the writer has complied with the general ground rules for successful writing the subsequent publication.

Successful writing and writing style is achieved and made possible by a thorough knowledge of the subject. Irrespective of prior knowledge of the subject, all successful writers spend some time reading around the subject prior to preparing a manuscript.

As soon as the manuscript is in its first or second draft form, give it to others for a critical review of the content and writing style.

Writing an article for publication requires practice. It is highly unlikely that any writer produces a perfect manuscript at first draft. Be prepared to write, rewrite and then write again before producing the final document. Be self-critical of all written work, and be prepared to frequently alter the material in the light of self-examination and advice given by others who have read the manuscript.

Participating in a writing workshop can be a valuable exercise, particularly for individuals who have difficulty in getting started.

Ensure that manuscripts are professionally typed prior to submission. A good secretary can give useful advice relating to construction and presentation of the paper.

SUBMITTING THE MANUSCRIPT

It is generally accepted that authors will submit manuscripts to only one journal at a time, this convention being widely accepted by journal publishers and by writers. Swanson and McCloskey (1986) report that the average time between manuscript submission and a decision being conveyed to the writer is approximately two to three months.

Following submission of the manuscript, one of three decisions might be made by the editor. These are rejection (with or without a reason being given), conditional, or unconditional acceptance.

Rejection

Letters of rejection may or may not include the reasons which caused the non-acceptance of the manuscript. If the letter contains no reason is for the rejection, there is little that can be done to establish what these are. Brosnan and Kovalesky (1980) suggested that helping to educate would-be writers was part of editorial responsibility. They suggested that, even when a manuscript is rejected because it is inappropriate for the journal to which it has been submitted, helpful comments could assist the author in preparing the manuscript for submission to other journals.

Whether or not the rejection letter details the reasons for rejection, the manuscript should be critically analysed and discussed with an informed colleague. If the rejection letter contains reasons, these should be considered prior to submitting an altered or unaltered manuscript to another appropriate journal.

Swanson and McCloskey (1986) asked journal editors to rate ten factors on their importance when considering whether to reject a manuscript. Although there were differences in the scores, editors of nursing and health care journals agreed on which factors were most and least important in rejection of a manuscript. (The most important factors are those with a

Table 14.1 Factors influencing decision to reject manuscript (adapted from Swanson and McCloskey (1986)

Factor (Average score on each factor)	Nursing journals	Health care journals
1. Content inaccurate	4.89	4.76
2. Content not consistent with purpose	4.61	4.68
3. Content not important	4.50	4.53
4. Content undocumented	4.36	4.45
5. Poor research design	4.30	4.51
6. Clinically not applicable	4.00	3.43
7. Poorly written	3.75	3.97
8. Subject covered recently	3.32	2.67
9. Content scheduled for future	2.86	2.61
10. Content too technical	2.12	2.53

highest score.) The editors were asked to rate the factors on their importance (1 equals not important; 3 equals somewhat important; 5 equals very important). Examination of these factors and their relative importance offer useful guidance in the construction and focus of a manuscript (Table 14.1).

Rejection of a manuscript should never be seen as indicating that it is not worthy of publication. Rejection slips are received by many writers who subsequently successfully submit the manuscript elsewhere.

Conditional acceptance

It is quite usual for journals to accept manuscripts subject to one or more specific conditions which are detailed in the letter of conditional acceptance. Examples are requests to extend or contract particular parts of the manuscript, suggestions that particular areas require to be rewritten for clarification or expansion, or the addition of sections which will make the paper more meaningful.

Assuming that you wish to comply with these conditions, the manuscript is altered accordingly and resubmitted. Should the changes meet with the conditions as set down in the letter of conditional acceptance, the progress of the manuscript is the same as for an unconditional acceptance.

Unconditional acceptance

Unconditional acceptance of the manuscript is, in fact, often accompanied by an indication that the editor will expect you to comply with *minor* editorial suggestions. However, as the phrase implies, unconditional acceptance of the manuscript will not involve significant changes. Additionally, the editor will send you a contract which contains two basic elements. First, the contract agrees that the journal will publish the article and will ask you to confirm that it has not been accepted by any other journal for publication. Second, the contract states the payment (if any) which will be made to you after publication.

AWAITING PUBLICATION

The time taken by journals to publish accepted manuscripts varies from two to fifteen months. Some weeks prior to publication, writers receive a copy of the galley proof which may or may not contain minor alterations to the original manuscript. The writer is requested to read and approve the manuscript before returning it to the journal for publication.

FOLLOWING PUBLICATION

Following publication, there may be little for you to do apart from enjoy that achievement. Occasionally, however, the article might prompt public discussion via the 'letters pages' of the journal in which it appeared. Very occasionally, writers respond to these comments by replying to them in the letters column of the journal.

MYTHS AND REALITIES OF WRITING FOR PUBLICATION

Myth: Writing for publication requires skills which are fundamentally different to those acquired during initial training and subsequent experience.

REALITY: The skills required for both types of writing are virtually identical, with 'normal' writing ability being easily adapted to conform to publishers' requirements.

Myth: Many 'ordinary' nurses have little to write about which is of interest to the profession generally, or to specialists in that particular area.

REALITY: *All* nurses, in all specialties, have the potential to make a useful contribution to the nursing literature.

Myth: Journals already have a sufficiently large number of submitted manuscripts from which to choose.

REALITY: Professional nursing journals would welcome a large increase in the number of submitted manuscripts.

Myth: Only 'senior' members of the profession contribute (or should contribute) to the professional literature.

REALITY: *All* professional nurses have an obligation to contribute to nursing knowledge via published materials.

Myth:　　　Successful writers have their manuscripts accepted on first submission to a professional journal.

REALITY:　Many writers (including those with an established published record) receive rejection slips.

Myth:　　　A good writing style is an essential prerequisite for getting materials published.

REALITY:　Although important, a good writing style is not the most important factor. More essential factors include the generation of interesting subject matter, the logical construction of the paper, and a clear presentation of new ideas (Table 14.1).

REFERENCES

Brosnan, J. and Kovalesky, A. (1980) As the authors see it. *Nursing Outlook*, **28**(11), 688–90.

Clayton, B. and Boyle, K. (1981) The refereed journal: Prestige in professional publication. *Nursing Outlook*, **29**(9), 531–4.

Cormack, D. (1984) *Writing for Nursing and Allied Professions*, Blackwell, Oxford.

Styles, M. (1978) Why publish? *Image*, **10**(2), 28–32.

Swanson, E. and McCloskey , J. (1986) Publishing opportunities for nurses, *Nursing Outlook*, **34**(5), 227–35.

Vivas, M. (1982) Getting into print. *Nursing Outlook*, **30**(8), 484.

White, J. (1987) The journal publication process: the perspective of the nurse author. *Journal of Advanced Nursing*, **12**, 121–7.

Wooley, A. and Hatcher, B. (1986) Teaching students to write for publication. *Journal of Nursing Education*, **25**(7), 300–1.

FURTHER READING

Bush, J. (1986) Seven steps from idea to print. *Nursing Success Today*, **3**(8), 14–6.

Campo, E., Pollack, L. and Hall, J. (1985) Tell the world your ideas. *Nursing Success Today*, **2**(2), 13–7.

Cormack, D. (1986) Writing a research article. *Nurse Education Today*, **6**(2), 64–8.

Duffy, K. (1985) Give publishing a try. *A.O.R.N., Association of Operating Room Nurses*, **42**(2), 230–4.

Hagemaster, J. and Kerrins, K. (1984) Six easy steps to publishing. *Nurse Educator*, **9**(4), 32–4.

Johnson, S. (1982) Selecting a journal. *Nursing and Health Care*, **3**, 258–63.

Kearns, P. (1986) How the nursing process can turn you into a writer. *Registered Nurse*, **49**(10), 10–3.

Methven, R. (1988) The book review; an education tool. *Midwifery*, **4**, 133–7.

Morris, S. (1988) Writing for publication: writing a book. *Midwifery*, **4**, 86–90.

Pinkava, B. and Haviland, C. (1984) Teaching writing and thinking skills. *Nursing Outlook*, **32**(5), 270–2.

Weinstein, S. (1986) Writing for publication. *N.I.T.A., Journal of the National Intravenous Therapy Association*, **9**(6), 469–73.

Wisenbaker, S. (1985) Writing for popular publication, *Nursing Success Today*, **2**(11), 5–7.

Sexton, D. (1982) Developing skills in grant writing. *Nursing Outlook*, **30**(1), 31–8.
Young, P. (1987) Writing for publication — an open letter from an editor to future authors. *Intensive Care Nursing*, **2**(4), 170–5.
Young, P. (1987) Writing for publication. *Nurse Education Today*, **7**, 285–8.

Chapter 15

Travel scholarships
DESMOND CORMACK

The considerable number of travel scholarships, sometimes referred to as travel fellowships, made available to health care staff in recent years offers an excellent opportunity for developing a career in a unique way.

The scholarships discussed in this chapter are those which enable people to travel (usually abroad) to study, or participate in, a well-defined area of health care. For example, they may enable a visit to centres of excellence in another country to study the structure and organization of multidisciplinary health care research, the care of the demented person, or the use of information technology in clinical nursing. Although all can benefit from this type of experience, some nurses may not be fully aware of the range of opportunities which exist, and many never consider applying. Given the large numbers of nurses, and the relatively small number of available scholarships, the competition is great.

TRAVEL SCHOLARSHIP PROVISION

Travel scholarship provision ranges from the local one in which staff members of a hospital or region are eligible, to the large-scale national or international one with a much wider eligibility. The small-scale scholarship may fund one person per year, the large may have resources to fund tens of applicants. A few organizations use part of their general health care, teaching, management or research budget to fund scholarships. Some obtain their income from charitable donations, others are part of a commercial organization. In all cases, the funding organization seeks to contribute to the development of nursing and of individual nurses, or to increase the quality of care received by a particular patient group. In part, the recent rapid increase in the availability of travel scholarships has been prompted by recognition of the internationalism of nursing and the way in which many of its features can be easily transferred between countries. Another reason is an awareness of the high financial cost of such an exchange of knowledge, ideas and skills.

Information about travel scholarships

Because of the expanding and changing nature of travel scholarship provision, no attempt will be made to discuss the specific ones which are available. Different groups of staff have access to varied types of scholarships and personal needs and eligibility will change with time. However, there are some general guidelines which may be helpful in indicating the range of possibilities.

Local sources of information

Those scholarships which relate only to a small group such as staff working in specific hospital or region are usually advertised locally. Information may be circulated via the line management structure, placed on notice boards, or made available to the local branch of the trade union or professional organization.

The professional press

Professional journals are the best source of information regarding scholarships available to a wide (national rather than local) group. The announcement may take the form of an advertisement inviting applications, be 'buried' in a news item or presented as a minor item of information. Examining back copies of a range of journals relating to the particular discipline, will 'give the feel' of where the material tends to appear. Because some scholarships are multidisciplinary or are international in their eligibility, the journals of other health care professions should be looked at, and those of the particular discipline published overseas.

Many newspapers and journals published by trade unions and professional organizations carry scholarship announcements. Membership of these bodies guarantees access to their publications; additional material may be available from librarians or from colleagues.

The popular press

A small number of funding bodies advertise in the popular press, these are usually scholarships available to the public generally, including nurses. For example, one major funding body in the UK advertises a number of scholarship subject categories in the national press each year. The categories, which may or not be relevant to health care staff, might include 'sewage disposal', 'crime prevention' or 'inner city architecture'. Quite often, the subjects include those of considerable relevance to nurses. Examples include 'diet and health', 'care of the elderly' 'prevention of drug abuse'.

Three major considerations are made when thinking about applying for travel scholarships. First, consider whether or not the scholarship requirements apply to you. This can usually be established from the advertisement, or by sending for 'additional details'. Second, consider whether plans for personal career development include foreign study tours at this stage. If you still have much to learn locally, or elsewhere in the country, do not be tempted to expand your horizons to the international scene too quickly. Third, consider whether personal and occupational circumstances will permit you to undertake a travelling scholarship.

It will assist the application if it can be demonstrated that your employer is supporting it, and by indicating how time will be made available. Three weeks of vacation time might be used, plus three weeks paid leave of absence from work for example. Alternatively, you might persuade your employer to provide a letter indicating that they will provide the full six weeks leave of absence.

The application

Prior to actually applying for a scholarship, there are important prelimi-naries which will improve the chances of the application being successful. Travelling should be considered as an extension of an otherwise well-developed career, sponsors will look for evidence of that development in the application or accompanying information. If you wish to visit coronary care units, be prepared to demonstrate that you are a specialist in that area, that you are familiar with the literature, that the subject is part of your present work, and that you are fully aware of local and national develop-ments. Be able to name referees who can confirm your expertise in the subject area, and indicate the use which can be made of the experience.

It is desirable, although not essential, that confirmation from a poten-tial study tour host be included, this will add much to the quality of the application and to the chances of success. This requires identifying and writing to the places you wish to visit well in advance of applying for the scholarship. My experience is that contacts in these places do not mind entering into a tentative agreement to accept you on the basis of 'should the application for a scholarship be successful, we would be happy to pro-vide appropriate experiences...' Such early contact with potential hosts may be made personally (providing you are fully aware of centres of excellence in the country you hope to visit) or via your professional organ-ization. In the UK, the International Department of the Royal College of Nursing provides such assistance (Banks, 1988). Clearly, this form of early planning must take place well in advance of submitting an applica-tion. The various funding organizations use a variety of forms for use in travelling scholarship applications. Typically, however, they will request the following type of information:

Curriculum vitae
The names of two referees

Details of the visit
Reasons for the visit
Supporting material
Estimates of costs (possibly).

A detailed curriculum vitae is included whether or not it is requested. This information will place the study tour in the context of previous professional training, experience and development. Funding bodies will wish to consider the extent to which the visit is part of, and an extension of, previous professional activity.

Referees

They may be asked to confirm the details of your application such as its relevance to your specialist area, and to confirm details of experience, qualifications, general suitability. As with people who provide references for other purposes, in support of a job application for instance, they are asked to provide a reference, and be fully briefed about the application. Giving referees a copy of the application, and all supporting papers, and discussing it with them is essential. The choice of referees is, of course, important. It is usual to name individuals who know you well, who have knowledge of the subject area of the visit, and are known to be supportive.

Details of the visit

The more precise you can be about the proposed visit, the better. Although successful applications may range from the vague 'To visit four well-known psychiatric units in the USA.' to 'To visit units A, B, C, and D...', I feel that the inclusion of more, rather than less, detail is much better. Ideally, you will have letters from the places you hope to visit confirming the availability of what you require, and their willingness to receive you. You will be asked to say how long the visit will be, and when you are likely to undertake it. You may be asked to estimate the cost of travel, accommodation, living costs etc.

Reasons for the visit

Funding sources are justifiably concerned that they only support applications who are using the visit to make a genuine contribution to their personal professional development, and to the work of their profession. They will expect you to provide a convincing argument in support of the application. Discuss how it relates to past work, present position, and to future activity. Convince them that this visit will enable you to improve your professional contribution, and that of colleagues with whom you will share the experience.

The interview

It is normal practice for funding organizations to interview a small number of 'short-listed' applicants. It is also usual for them to pay travelling and other costs associated with the interview, although this is not always so.

The purpose of the interview is to enable discussion of the application form and supporting material, explore further issues which are not addressed in it, and to enable the panel to 'have a look' at the applicants. In short, professional and personal performance will be under scrutiny. Be prepared to elaborate on any apsect of the material in the application. If you have said that you regularly read the literature in your subject area, be prepared to give detailed examples. If it has been said that Hospital X is a centre of excellence, be prepared to defend that assertion.

You may be asked to describe the use to which you will put the outcome of the visit. How will you share the experience with colleagues? Do you plan to publish a report in the professional press? How might you initiate change as a result of new knowledge and/or skill? Why do you think you should be given this opportunity? There is no way of predicting the questions to be asked in this type of interview. However, if the application is well prepared, the previous groundwork supportive, and if the application is part of a continuous and relevant career development, the interview should be present problems (see Chapter 19). In due course you will be informed of the outcome of the interview, success or failure!!

Being unsuccessful can be a difficult experience. Indeed, the fear of rejection probably prevents many potentially successful applicants from applying. Bear in mind that for each successful applicant, there will be many who do not succeed. Rejection may mean that the organization feels that you or the proposed tour should not be supported. More often, rejection simply reflects the limitations on resources. Many good applications are turned down because of lack of funds. Take a critical look at an unsuccessful application, and discuss it with your referees. It may be that it can be improved for use on a future occasion, it might be concluded that it should be used on future occasions in an unchanged form. If you have already contacted potential hosts, inform them of the outcome of the application and ask if you can continue to use their letters of support for further scholarship applications.

Planning the visit

If the reply is positive, there is much to do in planning the study tour. It is usual to receive details of the amount of the award to carry out the visit, this may or may not be accompanied by a request to submit an account of expenditure. It may be that all the funds will be sent to you on a specified date. Alternatively, the organization may arrange to pay major travel costs to your travel agent, and send you a cheque to cover additional costs.

Following acceptance of the award, you will probably be given written advice on how to plan the visit. Most major funding bodies provide excellent information developed from years of experience. Many professional organizations have an overseas department which is able to provide advice on all aspects of planning and undertaking a study tour. I suggest that you get in touch with your organization as early as possible and ask if they provide their service (Banks, 1988). Discuss the visit with your employer and confirm the previous provisional request for time off work if this is necessary. Set firm dates for the visit and get in touch with potential overseas hosts at once. See Emblin (1982) for further details of how to plan a study visit. If tentative arrangements have been made earlier, confirming these should not present problems. If not, make contact with the places you hope to visit, giving full personal details, and an explanation of the objectives of the visit. It is essential that you give precise details of the purpose of the visit, what you wish to do and see there, and how the visit relates to past, present and future work. Include the name of the sponsoring organization and, where appropriate, any special conditions attached to the award. Failure to provide the necessary information may result in delays in receiving a clear reply to your request to visit. Worse still, it may result in inappropriate arrangements being made. In due course you need to discuss arrival and departure dates, a timetable for the visit, accommodation, and to get advice regarding internal travel if you are visiting more than one place. In some instances, the services of an interpreter may have to be purchased or otherwise obtained.

Do not be surprised if hosts ask you to contribute to their understanding of the subject of the visit by speaking to colleagues in host institutions. They might also ask you to tell them about more general aspects of health care and professional education in your own country. Ideally, they should make these requests before departure, but this is not always possible, or it may simply have been overlooked. It may be prudent to take some written materials relating to your work, the health care system generally, professional education and so on. They may not be needed, but will help you to give formal or informal talks at short notice. Indeed you may offer to speak to groups of overseas colleagues; an opportunity to develop public speaking skills perhaps! (see Chapter 12). Another alternative is to prepare one or two talks prior to undertaking the study tour, these can then be presented 'on request'. The time required to finalize the arrangements will depend on a number of things including the extent to which you have, or have not, already made firm contacts with potential hosts. Visits to some countries, such as Canada, USA, and in western Europe can usually be arranged quickly because of the minimum formality required by their respective governments.

The visit

It is obviously usual for hosts to provide experiences (requested by you) which will meet the specific objectives of the visit. Additionally, they might identify other experiences which, although not specific to your objectives, are either related to it, or to your general professional background. The timetable should be sufficiently flexible to enable additions to be made. Following arrival at the destination, it is not unusual to be told about an additional person or place in the locality which may be of interest to you. If you are interested, ask if the timetable can be adjusted to make the additional visit possible.

Apart from the inevitable culture shock, often compounded by jet lag, it is common to experience a feeling of 'sensory overload' as you are exposed to many new experiences. These problems are made worse if it has been decided to visit many centres for short periods of time, rather than a few for longer periods. In order to maximize the value of the visit I suggest that:

1. Arrival in the country should be followed by a few days rest before starting to visit the hosts.
2. You visit less, rather than more, different locations in the country. My personal view is one or two weeks is a reasonable minimum period.
3. The timetable should contain sufficient 'free time' for rest, reflection and note-taking.

Be prepared to be exposed to a bewildering amount of new experiences and information; consider how you will record these. Unless you make decisions regarding this in advance of the visit, much will be forgotten before the tour ends. I have found a number of strategies of use. Some note-taking may be possible, particularly during meetings with individuals or small groups. However, there is always the danger that this will impede or slow down information exchange. Alternatively, you might 'write-up', notes at the end of each day, or at the end of each part of the visit during the day. The latter alternative will depend on having time available between meetings etc. during the day. I found using a hand-held micro-recorder of considerable value. Supplied with the machine, tapes and batteries, I recorded notes at the end of each day and, if the timetable permitted it, during the day between visits and meetings. Selective collection of appropriate documents, policy statements, care plans, publications and handouts of various forms from each of the places visited are a useful aid to the subsequent report writing. If such documents exist, but are not available during the visit, ask if they can be sent to you.

After the visit

Sending letters of thanks to hosts, sponsor and, where appropriate your employer, is done soon after return home.

Writing the report

Finally comes the inevitable, necessary and sometimes difficult writing of a report. Although the preparation of a report is almost certainly a condition of the award of travelling scholarships, it is also a means by which the visit is consolidated into a meaningful professional experience to be shared with others. The structure of the report can take a number of forms ranging from the chronological approach (starting with the first place visited, ending with the last) or be arranged by subject. In the latter approach, you might examine the material and identify and describe different topics irrespective of the time in the visit the experience was provided. Examples of the topics might be hospital care, community care, research, staff education; all relating to the main aim of your visit which might have been 'The care of the elderly with fractured neck of femur'. There is no 'recipe' for writing such a report. Be guided by the content of your notes and other information collected during the visit, by the structure which emerges from it, and by reading one or two reports which have been prepared by previous travel scholars funded by your sponsoring organization. A general outline for the report might be to consider and describe:

Personal details, and those of the sponsor and host establishment.
The reasons for undertaking the visit.
The aims of the visit.
How the aims were met.
Where and when the visit took place.
A description of your experiences, and of information obtained.
Interpretation of the experience and information.
Application of the material to your profession and health care system.
Suggestions for further contact between your country and the host country/countries and organizations.

Study tour reports must be written with a sensitivity and understanding which takes account of differing values, a variety of constraints and histories, and of the fact that you have spent a very brief period in another country. It is sometimes tempting to be over-critical of other systems, or of one's own system, following a study tour. This can be avoided by recognizing the limitations of the visit, and by learning from it rather than by making hasty generalized judgements based on limited experience.

Sharing the experience

Having written the report, you are in an excellent position to be able to adapt it for publication in a professional journal. This may require a condensation of the report to form a shorter item for publication as an article, or the selection of one or more parts of the report to form one or more articles (Chapter 14). Opportunities should be sought to inform colleagues of the outcome of the visit by making a copy of the report available to them, through individual contact, and by speaking at seminars, study days and conferences. In addition to submitting the report to your sponsor, seriously consider sending a full copy (or a summary) to your overseas hosts.

Using the experience

The visit will change the way in which you perceive your personal contribution to health care, and that of the profession. The new ideas, insights, information and experiences resulting from the visit will alter all future career development. The experience will also influence all those with whom you share it through publications and personal contact. The purpose of a study tour is not to enable you to immediately implement change on return home. The expectation is, in my view, rather longer term. Five years after the visit you may be able to answer such questions as 'How has the visit contributed to your career development?', 'How has it influenced your professional practice?' and 'How has the visit been used to influence your colleagues and your profession generally?' Perhaps these questions can be addressed as part of a career development evaluation a few years after the visit.

REFERENCES

Banks, A. (1988) Foreign exchange. *Nursing Standard*, **32**(2), 15.
Emblin, R. (1982) Guidelines for studying and working abroad. 1. How to plan a study visit. *Nursing Times*, **78**(30) Occasional paper, 117–20.

Part Three

Chapter 16

Professional options and opportunities

JULIA COXON

As we approach the last decade of the 20th century, nurses are faced with what would appear to be a bewildering array of career pathways. The decision about which route to take depends on a number of factors, not least experience. However, even newly registered nurses would be advised to think carefully about their future and according to Baker (1988) 'it is never too early to start to plan'. If experience has been gained in a haphazard way without planning it is advisable, and not too late, to take a long hard look at career and prospects. If you are returning to the profession after a break or seeking to change direction, you should also find a suitable avenue which will meet your needs.

POST-REGISTRATION TRAINING

On completion of training it may be that another course is the appropriate direction and the traditional pattern of general training followed by 18 months of midwifery has lost popularity over the years. There is other specialist training which may appear just as attractive and which will equip nurses to work in the clinical areas of sick children — mental illness and mental handicap. All of these may be taken as a first course or undertaken after registration which would mean the course would be shorter than for a direct entrant. However, with the implementation of Project 2000 and its implications for nurse education, the above pathways will change (UKCC, 1986).

Midwifery

Unless an applicant has first-level training (registered general nurse or registered sick children's nurse) then a three-year midwifery course is required. For registered general nurses it is a course of 18 months and a career in midwifery can lead into research, teaching or management. Opportunities exist for undertaking the advanced midwifery certificate or advanced diploma in midwifery. Midwifery is a qualification which can act as a springboard to work throughout the world. Whilst the midwife is practising there is a requirement for a refresher course to be taken every five years, an indication of the value midwives place on professional development. A midwifery certificate or an approved obstetric course is no longer a prerequisite for entry to health visiting training.

Community nursing

Recently there has been a move towards care in the community (Department of Health and Social Security, 1981). This report suggested that more care be offered in non-institutional settings, an admirable concept with which most nurses would agree. However, in reality, this shift of care into the community has not been matched by resources and the care is largely administered by lay carers, usually women.

Applicants to courses which train professionals for work in the community would do well to examine their motivation for such work. There is a difference between working in the warm 'sheltered' environment of hospitals, and to being out in all weathers, driving in icy conditions and carrying snow into the homes of the long suffering clients and patients. Just as special skills are required for hospital nursing, so different skills are required for work in the community. A practitioner who enjoys some degree of autonomy and can work happily either in isolation or who is willing and able to lead a team, may find community work suitable. Teamwork in the community differs from that in the hospital setting in that team members may be based in different geographical areas or districts and a positive effort is required to maintain channels of communication. Baker (1988) suggests that if a nurse is hurt by rejection of offers of help, or dislikes meeting with people who do not conform to his or her own views, then such a nurse may find work in the community frustrating.

POST-REGISTRATION COURSE PROVISION

National Boards publish annual lists of courses available to nurses who wish to work in the community. The major provision is in the form of courses in health visiting, district nursing, including those for enrolled nurses, community psychiatric nursing, school nursing and occupational health. Less well known are courses for practice nurses (general practice) and mental handicap (community). Usually, health boards or authorities offer financial support to candidates and, at present, this support is still forthcoming. However, recruitment is affected by factors such as manpower turnover rate and service demands. Many health boards and authorities usually make it clear that a *training* contract only is being offered, and there is often no guarantee of a position being available after the completion of the course. Therefore, you must give some careful thought before embarking upon these courses. Salary increments have not usually been affected previously. However, following the clinical grading review of 1988, it is worth taking note of this aspect of training. This should not be seen as an attempt to discourage potential applicants to these courses, but merely to urge you to think carefully when planning a new direction in your career.

In many areas there remains a shortage of community psychiatric nurses, but that does not mean individuals will be guaranteed employment on completing the course. That depends on the manpower planning and funding policies of health board or authority. You should take a written list of questions to the selection interview to enquire about turnover rates, manpower planning policies and other aspects of the post.

There are other avenues which lead to work in the community, some nurses opt for a further course of study to become health education officers or environmental health officers. The latter is an approved course which may be at degree level which is undertaken at universities and polytechnics and may be a lengthy process.

For those working in the community a variety of possible steps are available which may be in management, clinical specialization or education. Specialties in stoma care, counselling for patients with cancer, handicap, incontinence and contact tracing for communicable diseases are but a few options for district nurses or health visitors. Community psychiatric and mental handicap nurses may become specialists in 'portage' schemes or in alcohol problems.

The work of the occupational health nurse deserves special mention as this role can differ widely from that of surveillance, health maintenance and support, to being active in providing training for first aiders within a workforce. It all depends upon where the occupational health nurse works as to how the role is expressed. There is a difference between working as a medic on an oil-rig, and providing health care for the staff of a small National Health Service (NHS) hospital or unit. It also depends on how the company interprets the role and the opportunities it gives to the occupational health nurse to develop that role. Financial support for training in occupational health nursing may not be so easy to obtain and, in some parts of the country, it appears that the NHS is the main source of candidates to the course.

Many nurses will take the short courses available in intensive care, coronary care, neonatal intensive care and ophthalmology, information about these can be obtained from health boards or authorities and from NHS or higher educational establishments. Full details regarding post-registration course provision can be obtained from local NHS colleges, higher educational establishments and National Boards for Nursing, Midwifery and Health Visiting (see address list at end of the chapter).

NURSE EDUCATION

Those wishing to teach in NHS colleges or in higher education may do so by undertaking an approved course leading to registered nurse teacher. Alternatively, an MSc in education is a suitable vehicle to a career in teaching. First-level training is required to be able to embark upon such a teaching qualification. Registered nurse teachers may work in basic nurse education in general, mental illness, mental handicap or care of sick children. For post-registration courses, a midwifery tutor must hold the appropriate midwifery tutor diploma; health visiting lecturers must have a recognized health visitor tutor certificate which, at present, can only be obtained if the health visitor has previously completed a fieldwork teacher course. It is worth noting that there is a shortage of district nurse lecturers.

Working as a teacher in the community may be a reasonable career step. Fieldwork teaching (FWT) for health visitors and practical work teaching for district nurses is a popular option for experienced practitioners, a six-week theoretical course is available to prepare such candidates. The health visitor then becomes a probationer FWT for a further year (part 2 of the course). The work of the practical work or fieldwork teacher is very much teaching 'on the job' and can bring great rewards, it calls for dedication and high motivation as well as imagination and vision. To date, no such preparation exists for teachers in community psychiatric or occupational health nursing, however moves are afoot to arrange for a similar preparation to that for health visitors and district nurses.

At present, the clinical teacher certificate is being phased out and there will be one teaching qualification. Nurse teachers may take on a dual role of teaching in classroom and in clinical areas, or may have an emphasis within their role of classroom teaching or clinical teaching. Whether one opts to teach in basic nurse education or in post-registration courses, the aim is for all teachers to hold a first degree.

NURSE MANAGEMENT

At present it is difficult to offer information on a career in management as there is such a state of change within that field. However, nurses do attain top posts in management if they hold the right qualifications, a degree or diploma in administration may be the route to take. Information about these courses is available from higher education establishments. Nurse management in the NHS is usually provided within a line management system, and can have its rewards or frustrations. Perhaps the most important function is of support to fieldworkers. This is especially true in relation to managers working with health visitors and community psychiatric nurses. The support function in cases of child abuse or of violence is a vital aspect of the management role.

WORKING ABROAD

It used to be said that nurse training was a passport to the world and to an extent that is true. However, when a nurse decides to work abroad it is not a straightforward decision. Many considerations have to be taken into account, particularly whether to work and live abroad permanently or take part in exchange programmes; whether to work in western countries or in developing countries.

The elective

Medical students have for some time now had an opportunity to spend time in developing countries on what is known as the medical elective. However, Miles and Hicks (1988) discuss the possibility of nurses organizing their own elective. A number of organizations would be willing to recruit workers for a few months and place them with a long-term worker based abroad. Training is usually provided, and the organization will book flights and arrange other details. It is worth checking whether or not some degree of funding is provided. In addition, some organizations specify that workers going out on their schemes should be Christians. Informal links are another means of arranging a nursing elective. Having friends already abroad and also offering to finance yourself may tip the balance in your favour. It helps to be quite clear about your interest and, as Miles and Hicks point out, explaining your aims is probably a useful way of indicating that you are serious. Three routes are available when organizing you own elective, that of arranging a temporary spell abroad through an organization, or engaging in informal networking and finally in registering with one of the emergency organizations.

Voluntary work abroad

Careful thought needs to be given as to whether to work on a voluntary basis as this decision may well affect pension and incremental rights and bring about a net financial loss on return to the UK. In a pamphlet prepared by Returned Volunteer Action (1984), volunteers are urged to consider the full implications of the commitment required for voluntary work. They suggest that candidates ask themselves:

'Why do I want to volunteer?'
'Why am I in a position to do voluntary work?'
'Why are there people in need who have to rely on other people's voluntary labour?'
'What might be the effect on the local community of my working there as a volunteer?'

The above questions are designed to enable volunteers to think through their actions and to be quite sure of the consequences of volunteering.

According to Returned Volunteer Action, the majority of British non-missionary volunteers go abroad through one of the four sending agencies which are part of the British Volunteer Programme (BVP). BVP is a UK government backed body, 90% of its funds supplied by the Overseas Development Administration (ODA), which is the government body responsible for formulating and implementing British economic and social aid policies towards developing countries. The four agencies are: Voluntary Services Overseas (VSO), International Voluntary Service (IVS), United Nations Association International Service (UNAIS), and the Catholic Institute for International Relations (CIIR).

Much of the voluntary work abroad involves the delivery of primary health care in its broadest sense. Nurses may be responsible for advising on water supplies, crops or pollution. When asked what health project they would like to embark upon, the women of one village in North Borneo said they wished to embroider an altar cloth. The nurse involved did not question this but joined the women in the sewing sessions, much discussion on family health taking place during the sewing 'bees'. Subsequently, the nurse was able to introduce other topics and these were dealt with on a collective basis. This demonstrates how important it is to be flexible in one's approach. At the same time, you may be required for specialist work such as the care of people suffering from leprosy. Often, centres may be based in remote areas and if you are thinking of pursuing this kind of work you should have a level of maturity which will help you to manage culture shock and feelings of isolation. To know yourself and your strengths and limitations is probably the most important qualification. In fact, the United Nations Association International Service usually places emphasis on maturity and experience. They offer a minimum two-year contract, salary based on local costs, flights, accommodation, National Insurance contributions, medical cover and language training.

It would appear that opportunities for enrolled nurses to work abroad are limited. Countries prepared to offer employment usually employ enrolled nurses as aides, assistants and helpers (*Professional Nurse*, 1989).

Emergency relief programmes for overseas offer a relatively short period abroad and these are very much on an urgent or *ad hoc* basis. Many problems confront nurses who go out on these programmes not least that the aftermath of natural or man-made disasters tends to be epidemics of infectious diseases. Working in a refugee camp in the face of famine requires a special type of person. Organizations, which range from the lesser known to an agency like the Voluntary Services Overseas may offer sponsorship and payment, the latter at different levels. They usually provide workers for emergency relief as well as for longer term projects. The well-known agencies such as Save the Children, British Red Cross and Oxfam hold registers of workers who are willing to go abroad at short notice. It is worth noting that you may not be required immediately and may have to wait for a longer period before being called.

Nursing in North America

For nurses who wish to work in English speaking, western countries, North America is probably the biggest magnet.

United States of America

New laws on immigration have recently been formulated in most countries and the USA is no exception. However, because of the acute shortage of trained nurses there is still an opportunity for working in America. Several factors must be taken into consideration by the nurse who wishes to work in the USA. There are different requirements for working in different states, but most expect foreign nurses to hold the Commission for Graduates of Foreign Nursing Schools (CGFNS) certificate before being allowed to sit the State Board Licensing Examinations. A number of states require nurses trained overseas to hold a valid United States licence in order to practise as a nurse. Those desiring to work in the USA would be well advised to seek information from a professional organization such as the Royal College of Nursing, International Department.

Having decided to work in the USA it is worth preparing for the psychological impact of a different culture. Many people may find that their knowledge is obtained from the media and television in particular. It should be borne in mind that it is a vast country and Macilwaine (1987) suggests that the USA contains many states, city states, inner urban poor, and a super hi-tech first world. You should be realistic about these contrasts and about living in a country where the culture and standard of living is different.

There is no doubt that for British nurses, the USA appears to be a very lucrative proposition. However, those having worked there point to the high cost of living. In addition, American nurses feel they are not paid adequately enough for the work they do. Foley-Schmacht (1988) states, 'the money never goes as far as you expect it to'. On the other hand, White (1988) found that he managed to pay off his debts in Britain, and have a well-earned rest after only one year nursing in California.

Perhaps one of the most difficult areas for nurses getting used to working in the USA is actually doing the work. Foley-Schmacht (1988) states that nurses work harder and longer, but that the opportunities are greater. Macilwaine (1987) points to polarization in psychiatric care in the USA stating that on the one hand the care is excellent, but on the other it can be extremely low in comparison with other western countries. Similarly, she suggests that paediatric intensive care is the best in the world and that, at the same time, the United States have poor infant mortality rates in international league tables.

Contrasting views of the opportunities to exercise professional freedom in the USA are demonstrated by White (1988) who found that he had to consult doctors before taking the slightest action, and that of Yonko (1988) who found that written policies...and 'standing orders' gave the nurse parameters and freedom in practice.

Similarities between the United Kingdom and the United States are discussed by Trinosky-Lind (1988) and include nursing shortages with all the attendant problems. It may be that a nurse may wish to escape the problems she/he has encountered in the United Kingdom only to find the same problems in America.

Nevertheless, America has a lot to offer the trained nurse and Dunn (1988) states that: 'the USA is an incredible collection of experiences where the pace of life and stunning natural beauty go beyond anything seen in the movies....'.

Canada

For nurses wishing to work in Canada they will find that remuneration is very good and that nursing has a good public image. It would seem that, in Canada, education and autonomy are given greater precedence than in the UK, at least that is the view of Giles (1988). By the year 2000 all nurses in Canada will be expected to have degrees. Giles points to the changes whereby there seems to be an all out effort to enhance the status of nursing, in addition to improving the quality of care given by nurses.

Certain principles exist then for the nurse who wishes to work in North America and indeed in Australia and New Zealand. Make enquiries about the opportunities beforehand preferably from a reputable agency. Be well prepared at interview with a list of questions and enquire if there is an orientation programme before departure, and on arrival. Be alert to the possibility of culture shock and homesickness, keep an open mind and expect differences and similarities in practice. Most important is to seek advice from the International Department of a professional organization, such as the Royal College of Nursing.

Nursing in the Middle East

One location which attracts nurses and which deserves special mention is the Middle East. The remuneration for such work can be very competitive. However, this is but one aspect of employment and prospective candidates should carefully examine the package offered. What are the differences in clinical experience and in particular what are the pros and cons of cultural, climatic and social life in the Middle East? One needs to acknowledge and respect the rules regarding dress and other customs. The role of women is one area which differs from our western culture and female nurses may find the rules intolerable. Segregation of the sexes and the wearing of veils by the indigenous women are but two examples of custom which might be difficult to get used to. Relatives often stay in hospital with the sick family member and this is especially true of children. A great deal of tact and diplomacy is required in a situation where whole families visit the patient and where food, which may be medically forbidden, is a form of caring within families. Amidst the affluence of some Middle Eastern countries there may be third world features, such as dehydration, gastro-enteritis and an accompanying high infant mortality rate. Nursing in the Middle East has much to offer, but it is essential to find out as much as you can about life and work in the particular country of your choice. O'Brien (1988) found that accommodation and entertainment offered 'on site' led to a feeling of losing the sense of reality. Emblin (1982a,b,c) gives a set of guidelines for studying and working abroad and any individual wishing to widen horizons would find it useful to seriously consider such advice.

ALTERNATIVES TO WORKING IN THE NATIONAL HEALTH SERVICE

There has been a marked growth in positions outside the NHS and this is confirmed by scanning the advertising sections of current nursing journals. A few options are described here.

Prison hospitals

Prisons have their own hospitals which provide routine care and treatment. However, there is a variation in the provision of more sophisticated medical care. The larger prison establishments may have fully equipped facilities, whereas prisoners from smaller prisons may have to be escorted to local hospitals in the event of requiring specialized investigation and treatment.

Hospital officers in a prison hospital provide a link between doctor and inmate and as such have a challenging role. They are involved in preventive as well as curative nursing. For registered general nurses, at least one year's experience as a prison officer is essential before applying to become a hospital officer. The service welcomes registered general nurses, registered mental nurses and state enrolled nurses to their recruitment programme.

Nursing in the armed forces

Nursing in the armed forces is an area of experience where a dual role is in evidence. Perhaps the most well known is the Queen Alexandra's Royal Army Nursing Corps (QARANC)or commonly the QAs, where the individual is both nurse and army officer. A career in the QAs can be extremely rewarding and can offer variety as well as a challenge. There is usually an opportunity to serve abroad and the work itself is varied covering a full range of nursing specialities. There is also an expectation that, in time of war, nursing care will be required for military casualties. To be eligible for a commission in the QARANC one must be a registered general nurse with one year's post registration experience. Single, married or widowed nurses (without dependents) are eligible and the age restriction is 21–38 years. A medical examination is carried out by the army medical board at selection. Candidates must be British subjects or a citizen of the Irish republic in accordance with the nationality rules. Successful applicants are commissioned as lieutenants and subsequently attend a six-week QA student officer course at Aldershot. All new officers are commissioned for a period of two years, plus six years on regular reserve. The commission may be extended up to a total of eight years with a corresponding decrease in reserve liability. Specialist courses, as for intensive care are available. Although the word 'army' may conjure up an image of discipline and regimentation, the reality is that QAs have the freedom to enjoy a full social life. Compulsory requirements involve the wearing of uniform, attendance at training programmes which includes physical training and the occasional formal regimental dinner or function.

The Princess Mary's Royal Air Force Nursing Service (PMRAFNS) is perhaps not as well known as the QAs. The PMRAFNS requires applicants with a minimum of one year's nursing experience, to be registered on the general part of the register, and preferably have a second qualification. As with the army, those in the PMRAFNS have an opportunity to work at home or abroad and in well-equipped, up-to-date hospitals. Nurses working for this service also have the dual role, that of nurse and RAF officer. They are responsible for the provision of nursing care to servicemen and their families. Publicity material on this type of nursing states that RAF hospitals tend to be fairly small, with close working relationships and there is an expectation that nursing officers are involved in nurse training. Although single nurses may be likely to live in a bed-sitting room in the mess, they are free to find private accommodation off the station. How easy that is in reality is a moot point. Successful candidates embark upon a four-week course at the Royal Air Force college at Cranwell. First posting is usually to an RAF hospital in the UK. After four years, a nursing officer can normally expect promotion to the rank of flight lieutenant and after a further eight years to squadron leader, although this depends on seniority granted on entry. Suitable candidates attend interview and require evidence of medical fitness. They should normally be over age 22 years and not have reached their 30th birthday. Exceptionally, candidates up to age 35 years may be considered on merit.

The Queen Alexandra's Royal Naval Nursing service has similar conditions of entry, all entrants must satisfy the requirements regarding nationality and residence. They do accept enrolled nurses who must be between the ages of 21 and 28 years on entry. Registered general nurses must have had a minimum of two years' post-registration experience and be under 34 years of age.

Employment in the social services

The social services provide a wide range of care in the UK, with variations in how the service is offered within the four countries. The most popular option is to work in residential care settings either for mentally handicapped, the elderly or the mentally ill. There are sometimes marked differences in the way these residential establishments are run, with some providing a comfortable family milieu and others not so different from a hospital environment. Different levels of care are provided to cater for individuals with low through high dependency needs. Individuals wishing to work in such residential care would do well to examine their motives for moving out of nursing into this sphere, and if need be, make an effort to deinstitutionalize. Residents in long-term residential care are not 'patients', they regard the particular care setting as their home and accordingly need to be granted privacy. The informal atmosphere may actually act as a deterrent to such privacy as workers and residents may become too familiar. A criticism has been made that 'nurses' working as care attendants in the social services have brought with them hospital routines which were quite unsuitable for residential care (*Nursing Standard*, 1988). The social services may attract individuals who wish to work to a social model of health rather than a medical model; additional training may allow these individuals to become social workers.

Career steps into the voluntary sector may also include working in residential accommodation (such as a private home for the deaf), or undertaking salaried work for a voluntary agency. The latter may be a modest part-time contribution or a dynamic, managerial role as would be required for a director of a particular agency.

SPECIAL HOSPITALS

A special hospital is for patients detained under the Mental Health Acts who require treatment under conditions of special security. Special hospitals aim to have an active therapeutic policy which is undertaken within

a secure setting. Patients may suffer from mental handicap or mental illness. Nursing staff are part of a team with doctors, social workers, clinical
psychologists and occupation officers. Treatment involves assessment
(aided by nursing observation); acute medical treatment (including psychotherapy, drug therapy and other methods of contemporary psychiatric
care); rehabilitation (including social and occupational skills) and resettle-
ment. It can be seen that this is an area which requires specialist skills and
offers a challenge to nurses.

WORKING IN THE PRIVATE SECTOR

In the current economic climate the opportunity to nurse in the private
sector deserves mention. Swaffield (1988) reminds us that in the private
sector the range is very wide, the nursing experience on offer is varied,
and that provision is financed in many different ways. The range includes
what is provided by the voluntary organizations. However, nurses may
choose to work in acute clinical areas and it is evident that growth in this
sector has been rapid (Thomas Nicholl and Williams, 1988). According to
Swaffield nurses who decide that the private sector is for them may find
that: 'they have a public relations role they don't often have in the National
Health Service'. Usually, salaries tend to match those in the NHS although
nurses working for a private agency may find they can earn more. In addition, there may be fringe benefits and it is worthwhile for any potential
candidate to the private sector to ascertain what exactly is on offer.

Another aspect of private nursing is the concept of contracting yourself
out and offering skills in the market place as it were. In a so-called free
market economy this would seem to be a perfectly acceptable move. However, arguments about the moral stance of nurses opting to 'sell their
skills' may pale into insignificance beside the argument that nurses are not
equipped to negotiate and adapt in such an environment. This particularly
pertains to the suggestion that district nurses and health visitors could
contract out their services to general practitioners. To do so successfully,
arguably requires high level negotiation skills and a more equal power
base between doctors and nurses. This argument should not dissuade
nurses from getting into such an enterprise but anyone who believes the
market place is for them should carefully think out a suitable strategy to
ensure that they get a fair deal.

The nurse as an entrepreneur

For nurses with business acumen it may be that engaging upon a business
venture is a good option. However, as with any move it requires careful
thought and planning. In recent years the government has encouraged the
setting up of small businesses. The most popular choice, but by no means

the only one, appears to be the setting up of a nursing home and, with current demographic changes, there is a demand. Alternatively, you may wish to start up a nursing agency or provide a counselling service. All of these require a great deal of groundwork and as Holmes (1986) points out 'small businesses are known to be risky ventures'.

There are a number of courses throughout the country which provide training for those interested in setting up in business, and any potential business person would be well advised to attend such a course. It is worth obtaining information on the various enterprise schemes which would assist with the interpretation of law and would undertake the necessary planning. It certainly is not a venture to undertake lightly and Carr (1988) issued a prediction of a possible financial crash in the independent nursing homes sector. Whatever decision is made, would-be entrepreneurs should be thorough in their approach and heed the difficulties of making the business pay at the same time as providing a caring service.

A growing number of nurses are setting up practice in alternative medicine as acupuncturists, reflexologists or hypnotherapists. This involves not only business expertise but training in the alternative medicine method. Perhaps the most essential requirement is a belief in the particular aspect of alternative medicine and a corresponding commitment to it.

Joint appointments

An area worth mentioning is that of the joint appointment as these would appear to be becoming more popular. Quite a number of nurses now hold a joint teaching and practice position. Wright (1988) sounds a note of caution regarding these and whilst he points to the advantages of such an appointment, he also identifies areas of potential conflict. He suggests that you need to be a skilled teacher, clinician and manager with the ability to be flexible. Main sources for conflict seem to be between roles, within a role, and in relation to the role set. However arduous a joint appointment may be it can also be an enjoyable challenge bringing job satisfaction. Joint appointments involving community nursing have also been described (Howden, 1985).

Job-sharing

Job-sharing is an area worth exploring especially if you have family commitments. Opponents of job-sharing point to the lack of continuity as a reason for not setting up job-sharing schemes. However, with proper planning, continuity of patient and client care can be ensured. Lempp and Heslop (1987) point to the lack of job-sharing policies in the UK, and it may be that nurses, midwives and health visitors should act as initiators and consultants in bringing the schemes into operation. By working out a viable plan which suits both of you, flexibility could be ensured which would allow you to practise and at the same time retain a commitment to your families.

CONCLUSION

Perhaps the most salient point to emerge from any discussion about career pathways is the fact that nurses have many skills. They have abilities such as management and counselling and many now have experience of computers. Development of these skills in addition to special interests such as writing may mean that the career market is even wider. Nurses do become specialist counsellors, editors, top managers, consultants and successful salesmen/women.

However, there are golden rules for any nurse wishing to carve a career or pursue a career change. Have insight into your strengths and limitations. Carefully examine any package, especially the aspects relating to your pension rights and increments. Do not be afraid to ask questions and be diligent in your groundwork, preparation and planning. Maintain an open mind, flexibility and positive attitudes and be prepared for culture shock if you wish to work abroad.

Finally, this chapter is not a definitive discussion on professional opportunities, but is intended to encourage consideration of options which exist outside the traditional modes of employment. The emphasis given to careful planning of career steps is intentional as, perhaps now more than ever, nurses need to optimize their skills and widen their horizons. Most important is the need to maintain an acceptable level of continuing education and to appreciate the need for on-going professional development.

REFERENCES

Baker, J. (1988) *What next? — Post-basic Opportunities for Nurses*. Macmillan Education Ltd, London.

Carr, P. (1988) Report on speech by Dr Carr, General-Secretary of the Registered Nursing Homes Association. News section. *Nursing Times*, **84**(43), 8.

Department of Health and Social Security (1981) *Report of a Study on Community Care*, Department of Health and Social Security, London.

Dunn, A. (1988) A bite from the big apple. *Nursing Standard*, **32**(2), 7–8.

Emblin, R.I. (1982a) Guidelines for studying and working abroad. 1. How to plan a study visit. *Nursing Times*, **78**(30), 117–20 Occasional paper.

Emblin, R.I. (1982b) Guidelines for studying and working abroad. 2. General information. *Nursing Times*, **78**(31), 121–4 Occasional paper.

Emblin, R.I. (1982c) Guidelines for studying and working abroad. 3. Employment conditions and contract checklist. *Nursing Times*, **78**(32), 125–7 Occasional Paper.

Foley-Schmacht, K. (1988) Living in America. *Nursing Standard*, **32**(2), 10.

Giles, T. (1988) Culture gap. *Nursing Standard*, **32**(2), 18.

Holmes, P. (1986) Going it alone. *Nursing Times*, **82**(27), 28–30.

Howden, C. (1985) Community links. *Senior Nurse*, **2**(8), 6–8.

Lempp, H. and Heslop, A. (1987) Pioneering spirit. *Senior Nurse*, **7**(2), 24–6.

Macilwaine, H. (1987) A lesson from America. *Nursing Times*, **83**(40), 45–6.

Miles, G. and Hicks, C. (1988) Broadening your horizon. *Nursing Times*, **84**(25), 52–4.

Nursing Standard (1988) Recruitment Portfolio. Nursing in the Social Services. *Nursing Standard*, **3**(3), 21.

O'Brien, J. (1988) A personal view. *Nursing Standard*, **23**(4), 6.

Professional Nurse (1989) Career Development, Nursing overseas offers an ocean of opportunities. *Professional Nurse*, **4**(5), 254–6.

Returned Volunteer Action (1984) *Thinking about volunteering?* Returned Volunteer Action, London.

Swaffield, L. (1988) Nursing outside the NHS. *Nursing Standard*, **23**(2), 30–1.

Thomas, K.J., Nicholl, J.P. and Williams, B.T. (1988) A study of the movement of nurses and nursing skills between the NHS and the private sector in England and Wales. *International Journal of Nursing Studies*, **25**(1), 1–10.

Trinosky-Lind, P. (1988) America's dwindling pool. *Nursing Times*, **84**(31), 35–6.

United Kingdom Central Council (1986) *Project 2000: A New Preparation for Practice.* United Kingdom Central Council, London.

White, T. (1988) Nursing the American dream. *Nursing Standard*, **23**(2), 40–1.

Wright, S. (1988) Joint appointments: handle with care. *Nursing Times*, **84**(1), 32–3.

Yonko, C. (1988) America the Brave? *Nursing Times*, **84**(8), 31–3.

USEFUL ADDRESSES

Royal College of Nursing, International Department, 20 Cavendish Square, London W1M 0AB

The English National Board for Nursing Midwifery and Health Visiting, Victory House, 170 Tottenham Court Road, London W1P 0HA

The National Board for Nursing Midwifery and Health Visiting in Scotland, 22 Queen Street, Edinburgh EH2 1JX

The Welsh National Board for Nursing Midwifery and Health Visiting, 13th Floor, Pearl Assurance House, Greyfriars Street, Cardiff CF1 3AG

The National Board for Nursing Midwifery and Health Visiting, Northern Ireland, RAC House, 79 Chichester Street, Belfast BT1 4JR

The Nursing Adviser, Scottish Health Service Centre, Crewe Road South, Edinburgh EH4 2LF

The Chief Nursing Officer, Welsh Office, Cathays Park, Cardiff CF1 3NQ

The Nursing and Health Service Careers Centre, 121 Edgware Road, London W2 2HX

Red Cross, 9 Grosvenor Crescent, London SW1X 7EJ

Oxfam, Oxford House, 274 Banbury Road, Oxford OX2 7DZ

Save The Children Fund, Mary Datchelor House, 17 Grove Lane, Camberwell, London SE5 8RD

Voluntary Services Overseas, Enquiries Unit, 9 Belgrave Square, London SW1X 8P

United Nations International Service, 3 Whitehall Court, London SW1A 2EL

International Voluntary Service, 53 Regent Road, Leicester LE1 6YL

Catholic Institute for International Relations, 22 Coleman Fields, London N1 7AF

Methodist Church Overseas Division, 25 Marylebone Road, London NW1 5JR

BNA International, 470 Oxford Street, London W1N OHQ

Overseas Development Administration, Eland House, Stag Place, London SW1E 5DH

Returned Volunteer Action, 1 Amwell Street, London EC1R 1UL

The Health Education Authority, 78 New Oxford Street, London WC1A 1AH

RCN Research Society, 20 Cavendish Square, London W1M OAB

Distance Learning Centre, Southbank Polytechnic, PO Box 310, London SW4 9RZ

Head of Department of Nursing Studies, University of Edinburgh, Adam Ferguson Building, George Square, Edinburgh

Ministry of Defence, DNS (RAF), Room 704, First Avenue House, High Holborn, London WC1V 6HE

QARANC Liaison Colonel, Ministry of Defence (Army), DAR2. Room 1113, Empress State Building, Lillie Road, London SW6 1TR

Matron-in-Chief, QARNNS, First Avenue House, High Holborn, London WC1V 6HE

Registered Nursing Homes Association, 75 Portland Place, London W1N 4AN

The Head of Nursing Services, Medical Directorate, Prison Department, Portland House, London SW1 E5X

Chapter 17

Curriculum vitae preparation
DESMOND CORMACK

The curriculum vitae (CV) is a summary of biographical detail and of professional training, experience, continuing education and relevant activity. It is an overview of professional career development. Apart from personal detail such as name and age, the contents of a CV start on entry as a student, includes experiences before and after training, and continues to grow as a professional career matures. The 'richness' of a CV depends on the way in which you have managed your career. If you have sought out opportunities to develop your career, your CV will reflect that development; if you have been less active, your CV will contain fewer recent entries.

A CV which is often used in association with an application form, enables you to present a 'shop window' of professional accomplishments.

The importance of a CV has increased in recent years, particularly as geographical occupational mobility has resulted in many of us being unknown to those we wish to inform of our skills, experience and accomplishments for a variety of reasons. During the past few years, a number of commercial organizations have constructed businesses around the 'CV market'. You send them details of your professional background and they supply a well prepared CV — for a price of course. With the assistance of an able typist, and some knowledge of how to construct a CV, there is no reason why you should not do the job personally.

Curriculum vitae or résumé?

Although the two terms are frequently used interchangeably, some writers regard the two as being different; a resumé being sometimes regarded as a summary of a CV. I will focus on the construction of a CV and say a little at the end of this section regarding how it can be used to compile a resumé.

Gathering the material

All material relating to your professional career development should be summarized and written down as it occurs. For example, record the types and duration of clinical experiences associated with initial training, an outline of the training syllabus, professional visits, the title and subject of clinical and/or research projects, and details of any other discrete parts of your training.

Details of membership and use of libraries, membership of professional organizations and specialist societies, and participation in conferences, study days and locally organized seminars should be kept. Dates, and the content of all continuing education courses (however short) will be included in a CV.

In short, details of *all* professional experiences should be recorded as they occur. In due course, the record will save having to gather information five years after the event or, worse still, cause you to omit the item because details are not available, or are forgotten. This information, which will take a few minutes to record each two or so months, will make CV writing an easy matter. Additionally, it will be an excellent basis from which to undertake a career development review.

As your career progresses, the content of your CV will include less detailed description of earlier accomplishments and will focus on more recent material. For example, although detail of clinical experiences during training will be included in your CV during the first two or three years after training, this will give way to detail of experience following training in due course. Thus, the content of a CV should be seen as being dynamic and requiring to be updated with the passage of time.

When is a CV required?

A CV is required on any occasion when another person or organization wishes to make a judgement regarding your personal career development. In some instances, it may be the only (or initial) means by which you might be judged. On other occasions it will be accompanied by additional information such as that contained on an application form, or supplied by referees. Some examples of when a CV may be required are:

1. In support of a job application, in addition to details on application form, and the views of referees. I suggest that you include a CV whether or not it is asked for, and that you send the referees a copy as soon as he/she has agreed to provide a reference;
2. As additional material accompanying an application for a place on a course;
3. As background information when applying for a travel scholarship;
4. As an essential part of an application for research funding;
5. In support of an application for a higher degree;
6. When requesting that a professional journal consider you as a book or manuscript reviewer;
7. To meet the needs of those (mainly academic) employers who are

required to inform one or more organizations of employees' career development;

8. When being considered as an external examiner to an academic course.

Constructing a curriculum vitae

Consider having a 'master' record of professional activity from which to select material for specific purposes. Although this will involve the production of a 'new' CV on each occasion it is required, it is not something which needs to be done more than one or twice a year. The content should be determined by the specific reason for the CV request. It may be that the contents of a CV suit a variety of purposes. However, consider each item and ask the question; 'Should it be left in or taken out on this particular occasion?' Additionally, consider each item in terms of the amount of detail it requires; elaboration or summarization.

The presentation of a CV in terms of grammar, spelling, general presentation and attractiveness should be perfect. The work should be typed by a professional secretary, unless you have access to a word processor with which anyone can produce perfect typescript. If a photocopy is being sent off, it should be clear and closely resemble the original. Unfortunately, a badly presented CV can detract considerably from a high quality of content. Use of a word processor makes for easy updating of the CV and can result in an excellent presentation in terms of high quality visual presentation.

There is no standard format for CV presentation. Some institutions/ organizations may suggest that staff use a particular format, many have no such guidelines. A possible structure which may be used to develop a personal style of CV presentation is offered. The words which are printed in italics are examples of what might actually appear in the CV the non-italicized words are illustrative comments and would not appear in the CV.

Curriculum vitae

Personal details

Name
Home address
Home telephone
Work address
Work telephone
Citizenship
Date of birth
Present work position

At this point only include the name of the position (e.g. staff nurse) and the place of employment. When present work position is included in the body of the CV, it will be necessary to give an outline of the major responsibilities of position.

Educational qualifications

This section, which is in chronological order, will contain a brief description of professional and academic education. For example, the first three entries might be:

> *Registered General Nurse: District General Hospital School of Nursing, Leecastle, England. 1979–1982.*
> *Diploma In Clinical Teaching: :Leecastle Polytechnic, England. 1979–1981.*
> *BSc(Nursing) part-time. Leecastle Polytechnic, England. 1983–1987.*

Educational qualifications obtained at school have not been included here. However, if you are a relatively inexperienced nurse applying for a job, or entry to a course where such qualifications are important, then they must be included. This point underlines the fact that each individual must make decisions regarding some aspects of CV content and structure.

Clinical appointments

Also in chronological order, this section will provide a brief description of all clinical appointments. For example:

> *Staff Nurse: July 1982–January 1988. Smithtown General Hospital, Smithtown, England.*

Here, decide whether or not to include further details, for example, you may wish to indicate that the time was distributed equally between medical and surgical ward work. Such additional information will be necessary if you are a staff nurse applying for a sister's position in a medical or surgical ward.

The list of clinical appointments continues until you include your present position.

Teaching appointments

This section will be of relevance to staff who are already working as teachers/lecturers. An example of an entry might be:

> *Nurse Teacher: August 1988–September 1989. College of Nursing, Smithtown Hospital, England.*

You must then decide whether or not to include a summary of the major subject areas in which you taught. If you are applying for a first teaching appointment, or for a place on a teaching course, consider using an alternative sub-heading (*Teaching experience*). Items which could be included here are responsibilities for teaching learners in clinical areas, contributions to in-service education, and visiting lectureships at schools/colleges of nursing.

Continuing education

This part will include participation in all courses, study days, conferences, study visits etc., other than those which have been included under Educational qualifications. Unless a note is kept of these items as they occur, you risk overlooking them in a CV. Make a decision regarding how far back this entry should go. If, for example, you are a recently qualified staff nurse, then include all relevant experiences. Alternatively, if you have been nursing for many years, consider including material going back only five years for example, and stating this at the start of the section.

All information should be recorded and retained, you can then go back as far as is necessary for a particular situation. Bear in mind that, in due course, you may find it necessary to describe study day attendance which occurred twenty years ago.

Examples of entries in this section might be:

Conference attendance:	*'Nursing ethics'. University of Clarkstone. July 1st 1985.*
	'Advances in surgical nursing'. Altry General Hospital. January 19th 1987.
Short course attendance:	*'Infection control'. Netherfield Health Centre. June 18th–24th 1987.*
Professional visits:	*Paediatric surgical unit. Altry General Hospital. August 1st 1988.*

Papers presented

A full reference to each paper presented as part of a conference, study day or seminar, should be included. Examples of entries in this section are:

'The nature of nursing'. Nursing research conference. Warlton College, July 19th 1986.

'Anxiety in pre-operative patients'. Surgical nursing study day. Leefiled General Hospital, November 10th 1988.

Publications

A chronological list of all publications in journals, books and of published conference proceedings is a necessary part of a CV. If you are the sole author of the publication, there is no need to include your name at the beginning of the reference. Because many organizations distinguish between articles published in refereed journals and those in non-refereed journals, it will be necessary to indicate this. One way of doing this is by writing:

Publications (* = refereed journal).

Examples of entries might be:

*(1981) Making use of unsolicited research data. *Journal of Advanced Nursing* V.6, pp. 41–9.
(1984) *Writing For Nursing and Allied Professions.* London, Blackwell.
(1984) Editor *The Research Process in Nursing* London, Blackwell.
Unless instructed to do otherwise, all publications must be included in a CV.

Publishing related experience should be included under separate sub-headings, for example.

Book reviews.
Editorial panel membership.
Publishing consultancies.

Management experience

Because virtually every position, including those which are primarily clinical, education or research, include a management element, some reference should be made to this area. For example, a ward sister might write:

1981–1984: Ward sister, In addition to clinical responsibilities, management functions included those relating to (then include appropriate detail).
1984–1985: Relief nursing officer on two occasions for a total period of nine weeks. Management responsibilities were . . .
(then include appropriate detail).

Research

Participation in any aspect of nursing, or other types of health care related research should be included. Useful 'headings' for considering items are:

Personal research work.
Collaborative research work.
Research supervisions.
Refereeing research proposals.
Membership of research committees.
Research grants.

Awards and honours

Provide details of all awards which were made on a competitive basis, travel scholarships and research fellowships for example. Include a description of any honours or prizes. For example:

1976: Prize for distinction in surgical nursing. Forthfield General Hospital.

1981: Clarkstone Travelling Scholarship. Undertook a four-week study tour of surgical units in Swedish hospitals.

Professional organization activities

Active participation in the work of a professional organization is, in my view, an important part of career development. Entries in this section might include:

Member: 1970 Royal College of Nursing.
Chairman: 1975–77 Royal College of Nursing, Fairfax Branch.
Member: 1980 Royal College of Nursing Research Society.
Member: 1981 Psychiatric Nurses Association.

Other items which are be inserted include:

Consultancies
External examinerships
Committee memberships (past and present)
Workshop presentation.

General hints on CV preparation

1. It is prudent to assume that you will be required to produce a CV at some point, and that it will be sooner rather than later. A CV is a statement of fact which reflects career development. The better the career development, the better the CV.
2. Record information for inclusion in a CV as the events take place. Begin to record the details on entry into the profession.
3. Ensure the CV is well written and well presented.
4. Be consistent in presenting material in the CV, particularly within individual parts of it.
5. On occasions, it may be unclear into which section a particular item should be placed. For such items, simply select the section thought most appropriate. The important point is that all relevant information is included.
6. Prior to, during and after preparation of your CV, discuss it with someone who has some experience in this area.
7. The content of a CV is very often the subject of detailed discussion at interview. In preparing a CV take account of the fact that you will be expected to discuss, defend and justify every item in it. Also remember that you may be asked to explain the absence of particular items.
8. Do not regard the construction of a CV as 'optional' in that it may only be required by some employers/organizations. Writing a CV enables one to reflect on, and evaluate, personal career development, and to map out future plans.

The résumé

A résumé may be defined as a summary of a CV, thus, it would include all the major headings from a CV, but would present far less detail, for example, in relation to publications a resumé might read:

Publications

Six articles/book chapters published since 1981.

Similarly, clinical appointments might be summarized as:

Clinical appointments

1972–1986 Various appointments as staff nurse and ward sister in general nursing areas.

When asked for a CV, it is quite clear that a full CV is required. If a résumé is requested, I suggest that you clarify what is actually required; is it a CV or a summary of your CV? (a résumé). I include this word of caution in the certain knowledge that many use the term 'resumé' when they actually mean CV. If in doubt as to whether a CV or a resumé is required, send the latter.

FURTHER READING

Baker, J. (1989) Preparing a curriculum vitae. *Nursing Times*, **85**(24), 56–8.
Ellis, J. (1985) Getting a job: How to present a curriculum vitae. *British Journal of Hospital Medicine*, **34**(4), 237–9.
Fuller, E. (1986) Preparing a curriculum vitae. *Journal of Professional Nursing*, **2**(4), 201 and 266.
Gay, J. and Edgil, A. (1985) Is your curriculum vitae or résumé working for you? *Imprint*, **32**(5), 9–13.
O'Connor, P. (1984) Résumés: Opening the door. *Nursing Economics*, **2**(6), 428–31.
Place, B. (1988) How to augment your curriculum vitae. *Nursing Standard*, **18**(3), 39.
Sommers, M. and Sommers, J. (1983) Writing the nursing curriculum vitae. *Critical Care Nurse*, **3**(6), 100–4.

Chapter 18

Job search and application

DESMOND CORMACK

Virtually all nurses apply for a job at least once in a working life-time. This chapter discusses the means by which you might search and apply for a job, and to give some structure to that process. More importantly, it will place job search and application in the context of career development generally.

Most frequently, this activity will apply to those who are seeking one or more job changes in their career for reasons which may include changed domestic circumstances, and the wish to widen experience, for example, moving from a large district general hospital to a cottage hospital in order to obtain that kind of experience, or to obtain promotion.

In all cases the means by which we look for and apply for a new job are very similar. Prior to undertaking this, it is essential that past career experience is thoroughly evaluated (see Chapter 7).

In this chapter a series of steps, which hopefully can be tailored to fit individual needs, will be presented. It presents a series of guidelines which may be useful. Figure 18.1 provides an overview of a structured approach to undertaking a job search and application.

There are a number of ways in which a job search might be undertaken, depending on the urgency with which new employment is being sought. One person might be casually interested in the prospect of another job should something appropriate appear on the market, for example, a staff nurse might not be actively searching for a job, but may become interested if the sister's position in her ward became vacant. Although such an approach to job searching does not coincide exactly with the systematic approach to career development outlined in this book, it illustrates that many of us are open to offers should the right position come on the market. More often, a job search is based on a conscious decision to look for a new job at a particular time, and for a position of a particular type which will fit in with planned career development.

REVIEW CAREER DEVELOPMENT PROFILE

A career review will give a clear indication of the point at which you should (ideally) change your direction in terms of seeking promotion, gaining

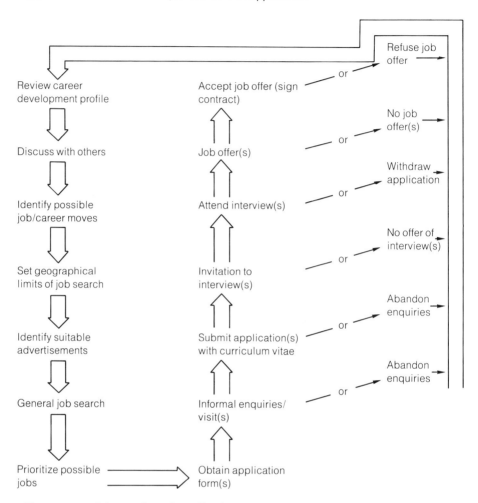

Figure 18.1 Job search and application.

further experience at the same level, moving into a different field of nursing, or into management, teaching or research. Implicit in this review is the need to answer two important questions. First, does my existing career profile currently offer the possibility for job/career change? Second, will I and/or a potential new employer benefit from such a change at this time? If you intend to look for a promoted post, ensure that your career development profile is genuinely sufficiently well developed to support an application for such a post.

Discuss with others

Much can be gained from discussing job search intentions with colleagues, senior staff or some other person such as a mentor who can be relied on to give an objective opinion and positive feedback. Similar discussions with friends and family will help to 'think through' the domestic and personal implications of making a career move. Although the final decision is a personal one, the support, advice and encouragement obtained from others can help in the considerable decision-making required at this point. The areas for such a discussion include the need for a job change, the type of position which coincides with personal requirements, identifying a job which fits in with personal career development and experiences, and the opportunity to discuss the advantages and disadvantages of a particular career move.

At this stage, a decision is made as to whether or not such as discussion will be 'confidential' or whether the information is to be publicly available to colleagues, present employers and so on. If the discussion is to be confidential, make this known at the outset. Clearly, success in this respect will involve a large degree of trust between you and others included in discussions.

IDENTIFY POSSIBLE JOB/CAREER MOVES

Recent developments in the nature and structure of the nursing profession have greatly increased the range of job opportunities. In addition to the well-established areas of nursing administration, research, education and clinical practice, many other career opportunities exist. There are also a large number of international opportunities in the above areas, and many new opportunities exist in the private sector, consultancy and publishing work, in government departments and so on. There is an increasing amount of interchange between nursing and other professions such as social work, psychology, the social and physical sciences, teaching, and personnel management. An examination of the job advertisement section of any major nursing journal which carries these will confirm that the opportunities available for qualified nursing staff are many and varied, and certainly not confined to 'nursing' in its strictest sense (see also Chapter 16).

SET GEOGRAPHICAL LIMITS OF JOB SEARCH

In recent years the international geographical mobility of nurses has multiplied many fold. Some years ago the only reason many nurses would have for moving from one country to another would have been to emigrate, probably for a lifetime. More recently, however, many are moving to other countries on a temporary basis, often as part of a planned career development (see Chapter 16). Geographical mobility need not necessarily mean working in another country of course. Decisions are made as to whether or not you are willing to move from your present location to another part of the region or country. It is as well to give some serious consideration to the consequences of geographical mobility prior to initiating a full job search.

IDENTIFY SUITABLE ADVERTISEMENTS

Most local nursing libraries carry a wide range of local, national and international journals which carry job advertisements. Some journals such as the *Nursing Times* carry a wide range of job adverts relating to virtually all nursing specialties at all levels. Also search journals of the overseas countries in which you might be interested in working.

Other journals are more specialized in the type of job advertisements they contain. The local press will often carry advertisements of vacancies, as will notice-boards in the work-place.

GENERAL JOB SEARCH

The next task is to systematically read through the job advertisement sections of the selected journals and newspapers. This is clearly made easier if firm decisions have previously been made in relation to job type, location and so on. Although most advertisements give sufficient information for a decision to be made as to the suitability of the job, this is not always so. If in doubt about the suitability of the advertised job it is usually best to obtain further information.

PRIORITIZE POSSIBLE JOBS

If a number of advertisements appear over the course of two weeks relating to jobs which may be suitable, try to place these in order of priority, considering their suitability from a geographical or specialty viewpoint.

OBTAIN APPLICATION FORM(S)

In some instances it may be necessary to request an application form and 'associated documents' in order to obtain fuller details of the position than were provided in the initial advertisement. There is, of course, no compulsion to apply for a job simply because you have obtained an application form. Indeed, you may be fortunate enough to identify a number of suitable jobs; obtain details of a few of them, and apply for more than one.

The additional information which accompanies an application form will vary from employer to employer. The following types of documents should be regarded as examples only. It is (unfortunately) somewhat unusual to obtain full information from a potential employer at this stage.

Application form;
Job description or details of the job;
Details of the organization and/or potential employer;
A general outline of conditions of service, e.g. salary scale, holiday entitlements, etc.;
Information relating to costs associated with interview;
A covering letter with details such as the final submission date for application form.

Further information of the type outlined above will guide decisions as to whether or not to continue with the application. In arriving at your decision, consider the following. Ensure that personal and professional background and experiences qualify you to apply for the position, and that you only apply for positions which are appropriate to experiences and background. Similarly, do not exclude yourself unnecessarily from applying because you think that you have little chance of success.

INFORMAL ENQUIRIES/VISITS

If the advertisement, application form and additional details contain sufficient information to enable you to decide whether or not to apply for a job, an informal enquiry *may* not be necessary. If, on the other hand, the advert seems interesting but does not contain sufficient information to enable you to make a decision, an informal enquiry (usually by telephone) may clarify these issues. Additionally, you may wish to pay an informal visit to the place of employment before deciding on whether or not to apply. Some adverts invite potential applicants to make such a visit, other do not. The absence of an invitation should not prevent you from requesting such a visit if you wish to make one. I *strongly* recommend that a visit be made prior to making an application (or after submitting an application but prior to attending for interview if selected). The reason for this recommendation is that the amount of time given to applicants selected for interview is very often less than ideal and rarely includes sufficient time for full discussion of the job, place of work and so on.

SUBMIT APPLICATION(S)

Although there are no standardized application forms, the following types of questions are typical.

Personal details represents a fairly straightforward part of the application form, and asks for information such as name, date of birth, address, present position and (possibly) present salary.

Full details of professional qualifications, with dates and where these were obtained, is also fairly straightforward. As with all other parts of the form, information in this section should be checked and re-checked for absolute accuracy. If requested, photocopies of the appropriate awards and qualifications should be enclosed. It might be as well to make photocopies at this stage in any event, as they may be subsequently requested.

Details of present position, and of previous positions with dates, names of employers etc. are usually requested. The normal practice is to list these in chronological order, giving full details of present employment and responsibilities.

Personal sickness and absence details are of considerable interest to a prospective employer. Whether or not this information is requested it is as well to have it 'at hand', particularly as it is might be discussed at interview.

Frequently, the application form contains a section which is titled something like 'Any other information'. To a large extent this section (in addition to an enclosed curriculum vitae) is something of a shop window which can be used to sell yourself to a prospective employer. Here, the applicant is given the opportunity to present additional information which may not be contained elsewhere on the application form. For example, it gives an opportunity to state why you are applying for this particular job. Additionally, you can provide enough information to convince the prospective employer that the job being applied for fits into personal career development profile and professional experience.

The names, addresses and professional positions of two or more referees will be requested. Because decisions regarding the selection of referees is one which is crucial to the success of any job application, this item will be discussed in a little detail.

Selection of referees

Potential referees can be selected from a previously built-up network of professional contacts (see Chapter 20). Possible referees are those who can be approached to discuss a job application, with whom you have had recent professional contact, who have the ability and status to comment on you, your background and the application, and (most importantly) be willing to support your application. In relation to the latter point it is essential that you openly discuss the job application in the context of your professional career development, and get a frank opinion from a potential referee with regard to suitability for the job being considered. If the potential referee has doubts about suitability, seriously reconsider whether or not to apply. However, whilst one such person may be unwilling to give a clear indication of his/her willingness to provide a supportive reference, you may wish to discuss the application with other potential referees and, if an indication of support is given, proceed with the application. In any event, submit the application only on the basis of having the assurance of potential referees that they will be supportive.

Clearly, the people who are asked to provide references should be appropriate from a number of viewpoints. First, they should be in a position to give a clear and credible comment on your suitability for the job. Referees may have worked with you in the recent past, or (less satisfactorily) know of your professional reputation at 'second hand'. Second, they should have an appropriate status and credibility which is acceptable to your potential employer. Examples of possible referees are the senior nurse with whom you have worked, the senior nursing administrator in your present or previous place of employment, and/or a senior member of the medical staff with whom you have had close contact. Although it is rather unusual for a nurse to give the name of a colleague from another discipline such as psychology or medicine, as a referee, my view is that this is quite acceptable if it is provided along with the names of one or more appropriate nursing staff referees. Third, one or all of the referees must have experience and knowledge of the specialist area in which the new job lies.

Having discussed the application with potential referees and obtained their permission to use their names, arrange that they are given a full copy of the application, any additional information, and a copy of your curriculum vitae. Apart from updating referees in relation to your background and recent activities, these materials will provide them with exact dates of employment, courses attended and so on. As the job application progresses, referees should be informed with regard to whether or not you are called for interview and, subsequently, the final outcome of the job application.

FOLLOWING APPLICATION SUBMISSION

On receipt of applications it is normal for a potential employer to take one of two courses of action. First, some take up the references of all applicants prior to drawing up a short list of those who are to be interviewed, others will only take up the references of those applicants who are to be interviewed. The nature of the short-listing procedure usually depends on the number of applications. For example, if 50 applications are received for a particular job, the best group of 3 to 6 may be selected for interview. Alternatively, if a relatively small number of applications are received, all applicants may be interviewed.

As is the case with those applicants who are called for interview but are not offered a job, prospective employers rarely, if ever, give a reason for not calling individuals for interview. However, if unsuccessful in relation to an internal job application, it is reasonable to expect to be given some indication of the reason/s.

EVALUATING POTENTIAL EMPLOYER

In the course of searching for a job, many factors will influence you in deciding whether or not you will submit an application to work for a particular employer, or whether or not to accept a position if it is offered. These factors are highly individual and vary from person to person. For example, crèche facilities may be very important to a nurse with a young family, whilst the availability of public transport may be essential to someone who does not have a car. Other factors such as staffing levels, quality of the work environment, and access to continuing/in-service education will be of considerable interest to all prospective employees. In the course of searching and applying for a job, identify and prioritize the factors felt to be relevant.

Just as the potential employer is evaluating you, you are making a thorough evaluation of the prospective employer. Table 18.1 contains examples of the factors which you may wish to consider in addition to those identified.

The answers to some of these questions will be relatively easy to find, for example whether or not the area is approved for nurse training purposes. Others, such as the level of multidisciplinary collaboration will be more difficult to answer. The only way to get a feel for the quality of an organization, or of a potential employer, is to visit and talk to people who are currently working there. Even then, the reality is that it can be rather difficult to completely determine the 'truth' until you actually go and work there. However, by thinking about, discussing, and looking at some of these issues during the time when you are selecting (and being selected by) a new employer, you will be better prepared to make the best decisions.

Table 18.1   Factors influencing decision to accept job offer

The job

General treatment ethos
Use of nursing care plans
Primary nursing
Multidisciplinary teamwork
Quality of patient care
Pay and conditions of service
Details of pensions/superannuation
Transfer of pension rights
Details of job responsibilities

Table 18.1 (cont'd)

Staff rotation
Shift system
Day/night staff rotation
Planned staff movement/development
Encouragement of research, publishing etc.
Evidence of staff research/publication
Induction/orientation programme
Promotion opportunities
Career opportunities
Job security

The organization

Management/clinical organizational structure
Written organizational plans
Ward/unit/hospital objectives
Management/employee communications and relationships
Quality of information available to prospective employees
Quality of interview/selection procedure
Quality of staff met during interview/visit
Approved for nurse teaching
Approved for medical teaching
Future plans for change/development
External reputation
Management style
Professional organization/trade union activity

The work place

Location and accessibility
Public transpsort
Cost of local housing
Staff houses, flats or other accommodation
Quality and location of school
Working environment
Relationship with local community

Staffing (quantity/quality)

Nurse staffing levels
Trained/untrained staff ratio
Paramedical and specialist department: e.g.
    occupational therapy
    physiotherapy
    dentistry

(cont'd)

Table 18.1 (cont'd)

---

chiropody
psychology
social work
recreational therapy etc.
Medical staffing
Size of wards/departments, and nurse: patient ratio
In-service/continuing education department staffing

Staff support and facilities

Housekeepers, clerical and domestic staff
Staff catering (day and night)
Staff library (up-to-date, staffed and accessible)
Crèche facilities (for present and/future use)
Information exchange; newsletters etc.
Staff meetings
Occupational health service
Continuing/in-service education
Provision/laundering of uniforms

FURTHER READING

Binger, J.L. (1985) Professional survival tips: Writing an effective cover letter and résumé. *Perioperative Nursing Quarterly*, **1**(2), 69–76.

Blanks, C. and Visscher, M. (1986) Organizational résumé. *Nursing Success Today*, **3**(11), 26–8.

Crossfield, T. (1989) How to...get shortlisted. *Nursing Standard*, **19**(3), 39.

Fardell, J. (1989) Selection: just The job. *Nursing Times*, **85**(21), 27–31.

Hurst, K. and Sakkal-Appleby, C. (1988) Getting psyched-up to stay. *Nursing Times*, **84**(43), 36–7.

Kershaw, B. (1986) How to play the application game. *Senior Nurse*, **5**(5–6), 46.

Larson, E., Lee, P., Brown, M. and Shorr, J. (1984) Job satisfaction: assumptions and complexities. *Journal of Nursing Administration*, **14**(1), 31–8.

Masagatani, G. and Grant, K. (1986) Managing an academic career. *American Journal of Occupational Therapy*, **40**(2), 83–8.

Purdy, E., Wright, S. and Johnson, M. (1988) On the right track. *Nursing Times*, **84**(39), 44–5.

Purdy, E., Wright, S. and Johnson, M. (1988) Change for the better. *Nursing Times*, **84**(38), 34–5.

Rose, M.A. (1987) Preparing for a job change. *Nurse Educator*, **12**(3), 11–12 and 38.

Rowden, R. (1989) Scouring the job ads. *Nursing Times*, **85**(23), 36–8.

Schober, J. (1989) Making a job change. *Nursing Times*, **85**(22), 32–3.

Shenton, H. and Hamm, C. (1988) How to retain nurses. *The Professional Nurse*, **3**(9), 360–2.

Chapter 19

Interview skills

DESMOND CORMACK

In the nature of things, some individuals are more comfortable, self-assured, and experienced in interview than others. However, I believe that panels take full account of any anxiety which some people *may* experience in this situation. Having been part of many panels for a range and variety of levels of jobs, and for other purposes, my experience has been that interviewees are rarely unsuccessful only because of their interview performance. The interview is a small, although important, part of a much wider process which operates in relation to job and other applications. The panel will place the applicant's performance in the context of the information contained in the application and supporting papers, the responses of referees, and general impressions gained during a pre-interview visit. However, one important function of many interviews is to determine the applicant's ability and confidence to interact with other people, and to deal reasonably confidently with pressures of the type generated by 'being interviewed'. Long-term career development, accompanied by making the right decisions in relation to applications, is a more than adequate preparation for successful interview performance. As with other professions (Hobbs, 1985) some nurses are not fully prepared during initial training for participating in interviews.

Interviews can take a number of forms and fulfil various functions. The primary purpose is to enable one or more individuals (the interviewer(s)) to meet with and talk to an individual (the interviewee) in order to evaluate competence in one or more of a number of areas, and clarify a variety of issues which may or may not have been addressed in an application form and supporting information, and to explore a range of new topics.

MOCK INTERVIEWS

I strongly commend those parts of pre-registration training which give interview experience to students who are preparing for a career in nursing, exposing them to a small number of 'mock interviews' which will prepare the way for subsequent successful performance. If this experience requires developing after initial training it can, and should, be organized as part of an in-service training programme, or form part of post-registration courses. Such a programme can give a fairly realistic exposure to what 'being interviewed' feels like. Additionally, it can increase confidence for participating in a first interview. Lee (1985) described a successful 'mock' interview exercise which could easily be used/adapted for use in initial training, or indeed as part of any continuing education experience.

INTERVIEW FORMAT

Most commonly, the interviewees and interviewers will meet in a more or less informal setting for a time-limited period. Although some interviews take place on a one-to-one basis, the usual format is for the interviewee to meet with a panel of varying size which will be 'chaired' by one of its members. Other interview types, previously mainly used for 'senior' positions (but now more often used for all types of interview) include the following:

First, the 'interview' might take the form of a group exercise where the interviewers meet simultaneously with a number of individuals who have applied for a particular job for example. In these situations, the interviewers are particularly interested in how each candidate performs in a group context, and on the person's performance on an individual basis.

Second, the interview might require the applicant to meet with a number of interview panels, each of whom look at a different aspect of ability and performance. For example, a job applicant might be interviewed by a peer group, by a group of administrative staff, then by a multidisciplinary professional group.

Third, 'interviews' in the forms of objective structured tests are being increasingly used for admission to nursing, and other health care courses (Jordan 1987a,b; Powis, *et al.*, 1988; and Walters, 1987) The use of such tests is, according to Hawkins (1986), becoming a feature of selection methods for many senior management posts.

Fourth, the type of selection described by Walters (1987) will, in my view, become more frequently used in the future. The elements of the multidimensional approach described by Walters, and in which each applicant was involved, were;

1. A traditional panel interview session with 'open' questions relating to motivation, work attitude and professional/technical qualities;
2. A second (simulation) interview which was designed to enable applicants to give an actual demonstration of performance in specific predetermined situations. Applicants were presented with a written description of ten common experiences and asked to;
   (a) Prioritize each of the activities from one to ten;
   (b) State who would perform each of the activities; i.e. you or another

person (if some tasks would be carried out by another person, indicate the position/grade of that person);

(c) State when the activity would be performed, i.e. in the morning, afternoon, evening or another day;

(d) Indicate (to the nearest quarter hour) the amount of time to be spent on each activity;

(e) Describe your role in relation to each activity;

(f) Write a rationale for determining your role in relation to each activity.

3. Applicants were then required to:

prepare a memo relating to a specific topic;

prepare an overhead transparency for a particular purpose, and prepare a three-minute talk on a specific topic.

Although widely used, conventional forms of panel interviews are of limited value in that they are too short, are a relatively artificial means of interaction, do not encourage relaxed and free communication, and cannot examine applicants' skills. It is probable that the comprehensive form of selection process (including interview) of the type described by Walters (1987) will be used more often in the future.

For the sake of illustration this chapter will focus on the more conventional type of interview in which an individual is met, with a greater or lesser degree of formality, by a single interview panel.

INTERVIEW FUNCTION

Although most interviews are part of a system designed to discriminate between a number of job applicants, they are also used for a range of other purposes. For example, to select applicants for places on academic and professional courses, for travel scholarships, or for research grants.

This chapter will address a number of issues which are common to all types of interview. For convenience, it will focus on the interview which is concerned with selecting one of a number of job applicants. All interviews (irrespective of format) are part of a wider process of information gathering in which the interviewers are considering its outcome in the context of a range of other materials. The additional information which is available to the panel, and which strongly influences its deliberations, includes the application form and additional material (if any), curriculum vitae, and the opinions of the referees.

Most interviews are well conducted and positively discriminate in favour of each of those being interviewed. 'Being interviewed' is an unnatural circumstance in which few individuals build up much experience. In relation to the panel, the interviewee is relatively disadvantaged and powerless. However, a good panel led by an able chairperson will do everything possible to maximize the performance of each candidate. The interview allows for further detailed discussion and exploration of a number of issues which are not possible to evaluate solely by reading the application form, references and other documents. It also allows for face to face examination and consideration of the personality, attitude and interpersonal ability of the applicant. This part of the selection process gives the opportunity for interviewees to 'sell themselves' in a way which is not possible in the application form or, indeed, in any other written format. The experience is a two-way one in which you are evaluating a potential employer, who in turn is evaluating one or more potential employees or other type of applicant.

PREPARATION FOR INTERVIEW

In the months or years prior to interview, appropriate career development will give a sound basis for maximizing performance. Continual and long-term involvement in the various aspects of career development which are discussed in this text are important pre-requisites for success. The least effective form of preparation is to invest time and energy in career development and preparation *after* being invited for interview. Indeed, such a preparation will probably result in a poor performance which gives little satisfaction to those involved.

In the period between receiving the invitation and attending the interview, there are a number of things which can be done by way of additional preparation. First, re-read the job advertisement (including the fine print) and, more importantly, read and consider every item in the job description. When reading the elements of the job description, consider each of its parts in relation to previous professional experience, knowledge and skill. Much of the interview will undoubtedly focus on applicants' ability to deal with specific items in the job description. Invariably, interviewees are better equipped to deal with some aspects of the new employment than with others.

At this point, consider strengths and *relative* weaknesses in relation to the new position and, where appropriate, be prepared to discuss these in terms of how any identified weaknesses (if any) might be 'made good', or compensated for by strengths.

Obtain the most recent general publications relating to the position. Ensure familiarity with the literature in relation to the demands of the position, read and re-read the documents immediately prior to interview. Study any local documents which relate to the particular hospital and/or position being applied for. These might be hospital newsletters, staff publications or policy documents relating to the hospital or the specialty.

A systematic and detailed review of personal career development profile is made, and the outcome compared with the requirements of the new position. This comparison will enable a realistic evaluation of particular strengths and weaknesses to be made.

The opportunity is then taken (if not already done so) to discuss the application with a colleague who holds a similar position to that being applied for, and with a mentor. This discussion focuses on personal career profile compared with the requirements of the new position.

If an informal visit has not been arranged prior to, or in association with, the interview, this should be seriously considered.

Finally, a short list of relevant qustions should be created and written down. Although the questions may well be modified at a later stage, it is as well to start thinking about this area sooner rather than later.

THE INTERVIEW

Clearly, interviewees are expected to arrive on time. In the interests of safety, and taking account of the possibilities of car breakdown and/or failure of public transport, arrive well ahead of time. Arriving late might result in no interview taking place, and will certainly cause a bad impression. Better to arrive very early and be on time and relaxed, than be slightly late or otherwise rushing there. Just as the interviewee will be expected to arrive on time you will justifiably expect the interview to begin promptly. Some interviews start later than scheduled, this occasionally being caused by the panel either making a late start to the group of interviews, or by one or more of the interviews 'running late'. Whatever the cause of delay, it is usually the result of bad planning, failure to keep to a timetable within or between interviews, or (more worrying) the result of poor work on the part of the chairperson. The need for the interview panel to be prompt and keep to an agreed schedule was underlined by Bray (1984) who observed that: 'The applicant will be anxious in anticipation of the interview, and delaying the process will only serve to intensify this feeling.'

Dress

In addition to nursing being a conservative profession in terms of the clothes worn by its members, interviews are a relatively formal event in which the interviewers and interviewees normally wear conservative clothes such as suits, shirts, ties and the feminine equivalents. Rightly or wrongly, most interview panels would not be impressed by applicants who arrived wearing sandshoes, jeans and open-necked shirts.

Interview documentation

Bring along a copy of all the documents which have been prepared in relation to the application: a copy of your curriculum vitae, completed application form, job description and other documents which have been prepared by, or sent to, you. Although these documents will not be required in all instances, they are certainly useful as a point of reference should a particular item cause confusion and need clarification. Apart from a briefcase or folder containing interview documents, I strongly suggest that no other items of 'luggage' be taken into the interview room.

Meeting other interviewees

It is not uncommon for a number of interviewees to tour the facility together, or be left together in a waiting room, particularly if the interviews are running late. Although some applicants find 'meeting the opposition' somewhat disconcerting, it need not be so. Apart from social and professional conversation, this waiting time can be used profitably in general discussion with regard to the job and prospective employer. It is also an opportunity to begin to get into the spirit of the interview, and to further rehearse how some issues might be addressed.

The interview room

It is normal practice for an interview panel member, or some other person, to invite applicants to meet with the interview panel. After entering the room, wait until invited to use a particular seat. Over-hasty selection of a seat might result in the slightly embarrassing position of sitting in the wrong place and having to be re-directed to the 'interviewee seat'. On being invited to sit down, place interview papers on the table and give a brief explanation such as 'I have brought my interview papers for reference'.

If the interview panel consists of more than one person it is usual for a member to take the role of chairperson or otherwise take some form of leadership role. Even if a list of the interview panel membership has been previously obtained, it is normal practice for the chairperson to extend a welcome to the candidate and go on to introduce the panel members. Although good interview practice dictates that this information be made available in advance, it is unfortunately the case that this is not always done. However, one consolation is that other interviewees are equally disadvantaged.

Following the introductory 'pleasantries' the chairperson will invite individual panel members to ask questions and/or raise points for discussion. Alternatively, the chairperson may personally begin the discussion.

INTERVIEW STRUCTURE

Before continuing with this section, it will be profitable to briefly examine the advice which is given to interview panel members by Beardwell and Harris (1987) who suggested that:

...each topic area should have more questions prepared than are likely to be used; within the total interview (including the answering of candidates' questions) the interviewers should not be talking for more than 25% of the time; the questions should be pertinent, expressed clearly and one at a time. A rapid barrage of questions, thinking aloud etc., only creates confusion; questions should be designed to provoke a detailed answer and not merely 'yes' or 'no'; each answer should be followed up so that each opinion, attitude or statement is fully aired. Never assume an answer — the skilled interviewee has the knack of leaving things in the air. The use of the words 'how', 'which', 'why', 'when' is recommended; an interview is in part a public relations exercise and the whole atmosphere must encourage the candidates to give of their best. Therefore it is recommended that panel members avoid aggressive inquisitioning and do not attempt to demonstrate to the other panel members that they have cleverly trapped the candidate. A clear aim of an employing authority should be to send unsuccessful candidates away feeling genuinely sorry to have missed the job as it seemed a good place in which to work (pp. 7–8).

This advice to interview panels not only illustrates how interview questioning should be conducted, but also some of the areas in which interviewers can 'get it wrong'. Prior knowledge of these possible problem areas makes them easier to deal with should they occur. Although considerable variation exists in the structure of interviews, the following structure is typical of many.

It is usual to commence with questions of a relatively closed type which serve to clarify some points of detail, and to put the interviewee at ease. Examples of such questions are 'Do you work in a male or female ward?', 'Can you tell me a little about the post-registration course which you took last year?' and 'Where did you read the advertisement for this job?'

Clinical

Clinical experiences, details of the nature and specialist content of previous work, and its relationship to the position being applied for will be discussed. You will be expected to demonstrate a current and detailed knowledge of the clinical area involved. It is also necessary to demonstrate a knowledge of, and familiarity with, recent published materials (including those which are research based). For clinical positions, this area of discussion will obviously constitute the greater part of the interview.

Management

Virtually all nursing positions have a management component which require competence at that particular level. The job description will detail the management responsibilities in relation to the position. These should be studied carefully in advance of the interview, and responses to relevant questions considered.

Research

A familiarity with, and an ability to evaluate, recent research is a normal expectation in relation to all nursing positions (Chapter 9). The panel will expect you to talk with some confidence on research-related issues, and to have some familiarity with the purpose, nature and language of research.

Teaching

Whether or not the proposed area of work involves teaching student nurses, all registered nurses have a role to play in relation to teaching qualified and unqualified nursing colleagues. A careful assessment of previous clinical experience will undoubtedly demonstrate that much time has been spent in teaching others. A few nurses unfortunately tend to overlook the many and varied informal occasions when they have functioned as 'teachers' in relation to fellow professionals and patients.

If the job description has an explicit component relating to teaching responsibilities, be prepared to discuss this in detail and to demonstrate how you might fulfil this requirement. If there are any doubts about this area prior to interview, it would be useful to discuss this item with a teaching colleague.

Career development

Although the application form and curriculum vitae will give a general overview of career to date, it is usual for panel members to seek expansion of details of particular parts of a career, and to ask how it will develop in future. Be prepared to answer this question from two perspectives; first, if the job is offered, second, how the career might develop should this particular post not be offered.

Knowledge of position being applied for

Undoubtedly, some considerable time will be spent on discussing the detailed aspects of the job being applied for. Be prepared to answer questions relating to any aspect of the post. Be prepared to state how previous training and career development have prepared you for dealing with particular aspects of the position.

In relation to the above general structure it is always difficult to predict the specific types of questions which may be asked. Indeed, some of the questions may be of a fairly general nature and be outside any particular part of the structure. The following are examples of the types of questions which may be asked and dealt with without much difficulty, providing that prior long-term career development has been undertaken.

- Tell us about yourself and your background?
- What prompted you to apply for this particular job?
- What are the special qualities which you feel you could bring to this job?
- What are your strongest and weakest points?
- What would you plan to do if you are unsuccessful here?
- How do you keep up to date?
- Which professional journals do you read, and give us some examples of the things you have read recently?
- How did you prepare for this interview?
- How do you see the future of nursing developing?
- What personal qualities do you feel have contributed most to your career so far?
- How do you see your career developing during the next five years?
- How would you describe your leadership style, and its strengths and weaknesses?
- Who do you regard as being the leaders in nursing generally, and in your specialty in particular?
- What if...(the interviewer would then describe a specific problem situation) occurred. How might you deal with this situation?

Many of the above questions are 'discursive' in nature and demonstrate the difference between two major types of questions which are frequently used in interview. The closed question is one which requires a short factual answer, e.g. 'Where did you work before you came into nursing?' An open question is one which requires a much more discursive reply, e.g. 'How do you see this job fitting into your long-term professional career development?'

It is usual, but by no means universal, that the panel members will use a list of predetermined criteria when asking questions and recording responses. See Battle *et al.* (1985) for an example of a structured interview/rating guide.

At the end of the interview, applicants are normally invited to ask any questions which they have in mind. These might relate to the job being applied for, conditions of employment, or the general organization in which the job will be performed. This item is discussed in more detail later in this chapter.

CONCLUSION

Although the outcome of interview performance can never be guaranteed (but it can be improved by an adequate professional career development) the following items may be of value.

Frankness

Whilst the main purpose of the interview is to establish what the applicant knows, rather than what the applicant does not know, it is quite appropriate for a panel to push interviewees to their limits of knowledge and ability to respond. Only by doing so can they determine the full extent of your knowledge and ability. Because of this, there comes a time in many interviews when a question is asked to which you have no answer. On such occasions it is probably best to respond by saying that you do not know the answer, and to go on to explain how one might obtain an answer to it. Although a panel would not expect to have many 'I don't know' replies, they will respond positively, providing you recognize the need to find the answers, and the means of doing so.

Accuracy

Responses should be an accurate reflection of experience, present position and, where appropriate, a realistic prediction of the future. Replies to questions concerning the future are, in common with all other material, often recorded in detail. Caution should be exercised when replying to questions regarding future intentions and plans, in order to ensure that they are realistic and can be met if the job is obtained. Rash or over-ambitious promises made during interview can come back to 'haunt' a successful applicant who, for any of a number of reasons, fails to keep these.

Participation

The purpose of all questions is to give you an opportunity to make a well-informed and assertive response. Questions of the closed type require a brief reply, while those of the open type require a more detailed response. In relation to the former the panel do not expect a five minute reply in response to a question such as 'How many years have you been in nursing?', nor do they expect a single word reply to a question such as 'What particularly interests you in this new position?' Judgement needs to be used in relation to the detail with which you respond to a particular question.

Assertiveness

Appropriate long-and short-term preparation for the interview will ensure that responses are made in a confident and assertive manner. Positive and constructive replies (rather than those which are extremely contentious and/or destructive) tend to be well received. In general, interviewers prefer responses which indicate that you have 'thought through' these issues and possible replies prior to the interview. *Be prepared to defend, justify and explain all replies.* Never assume that because your views differ from those of an interviewer, they are necessarily wrong.

Any questions?

I suggest that a small number of relevant and brief questions be prepared in writing prior to the interview. Additionally, relevant questions may come to mind in the course of an interview. On being invited to ask questions, feel free to refer to the previously prepared note of these. Questions should only be of a kind which could not have appropriately been dealt with prior to the interview. Bearing in mind that, at the end of an interview, there normally remains a number of unanswered questions, panels generally expect candidates to ask these. I am not suggesting that, in principle, such questions should always be asked. Rather, I am suggesting that the opportunity should be taken to raise these when appropriate. Seriously consider asking 'what do you have to offer me?' If the panel find the question unreasonable, or are unable to give a convincing answer, draw your own conclusions.

For those who have never been interviewed for a job or for some other reason, the prospect can be a challenging one; others who have participated in one or more successful interviews, reflect on the experience with a feeling of considerable satisfaction. The term 'successful' is not confined to being offered that for which an application had been submitted. Rather, it refers to feeling good about an interview performance, knowing that responses to questions were satisfactory, and to leaving the interview room with a feeling of having been fully prepared for the experience. Interviews can be approached with confidence when the participant has given sufficient time and attention to professional development. Indeed, a well-conducted interview, and they are in the majority, will positively discriminate in favour of each interviewee, with panel members doing all that is possible to ensure that candidates perform well.

REFERENCES

Battle, E., Bragg, S., Delaney, J. *et al.* (1985) Developing a rating interview guide. *Journal of Nursing Administration*, **15**(10), 39–45.
Bayne, M., Parker, B. and Todd, A. (1982) The search committee process. *Nursing Outlook*, **30**(3), 178–81.
Beardwell, M. and Harris, G. (1987) *Effective Interviewing*. National Association of Health Authorities, London.
Bray, K. (1984) The interview process. *Critical Care Nurse*, **4**(3), 65–7.

Hawkins, C. (1986) Trial by sherry. *Senior Nurse*, **4**(1), 21.

Hobbs, K. (1985) Getting a job. The interview. *British Journal of Hospital Medicine*, **33**(4), 220–2.

Jordan, M. (1987a) Safe selection. *Nursing Times*, **83**(43), 40–1.

Jordan, M. (1987b) Just right for the job. *Nursing Times*, **83**(42), 45–6.

Lee, D. (1985) A process of elimination. *Nursing Mirror*, **160**(7), 42–3.

Powis, D., Neame, R., Bristow, T. and Murphy, L. (1988). The objective, structured interview for medical student selection. *British Medical Journal*, **296**, 765–8.

Walters, J. (1987) An innovative method of job interviewing. *Journal of Nursing Administration*, **17**(5), 25–9.

Part Four

Chapter 20

Professional networking

PHILIP BARKER

INTRODUCTION

The social system of nursing is especially complex. Nurses are exposed to the range of difficulties met by ordinary people and to a range of professional challenges besides. Many of the problems met by nurses in their work centre upon relationships: their relationships with patients, colleagues and themselves. The solution to most of such difficulties is also to be found in relationships: special relationships which are invoked in an attempt to gain greater understanding. Nurses can use their relationships with one another, and sometimes other professionals, to resolve the relationship issues which are inherent in their professional lives. This chapter focuses upon how nurses can use professional relationships to resolve difficulties in their work and as a vital means of professional development.

People also need other people. The need to 'belong' is perhaps our most distinctive feature. The person who does not belong, or who feels that she does not belong, is powerless to understand 'her world', is alienated, and experiences the anomie or 'normlessness' described by Durkheim (1933). The 'norms', standards, values, or beliefs of our professional group are a steadying force in our professional lives. This chapter is about developing and maintaining the supports which give meaning to our professional lives. Emphasis will be given to four main areas of social support which nurses can use to aid professional development embraced within the concept of the social network. The chapter assumes that some readers will be interested in the roles of preceptor or preceptee. Others will be more concerned with learning from, or acting as, a role model. A third group of readers might be expected to act as, or may be interested in using the help of, a mentor.

THE SOCIAL NETWORK

Your social network is the collective title for the people and organizations with whom you communicate. Here we are talking about people whom you know who may, or may not, know one another, and who have the

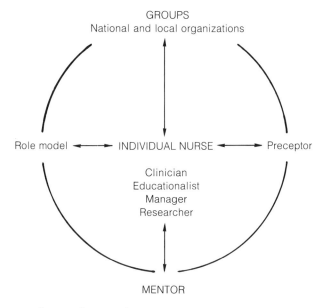

GROUPS
National and local organizations

Role model ←——→ INDIVIDUAL NURSE ←——→ Preceptor

Clinician
Educationalist
Manager
Researcher

MENTOR

Figure 20.1 Professional networking.

potential to help you to develop professionally. Your social network can be very informal, when meeting with colleagues for lunch or coffee, socializing after work, discussing your problems, ideas and general attitudes towards your professional 'self'.

More formal examples exist in organized meetings where you discuss or debate innovations in nursing theory and practice. You are 'networking' when you establish contact with colleagues, for the first time or routinely, with the aim of advancing your own, or others', professional skills or knowledge. This network is illustrated in Figure 20.1. Four main groups of people are embraced by your social network: role models who serve as professional 'examples', mentors whom you choose to turn to for advice or guidance, preceptors who offer support or guidance and various groups who provide alternatives to the other three.

Emphasis will be given here to the role of the network in developing the nurse's skills and knowledge. Most of the examples included refer to relatively direct forms of facilitation. In addition, however, your social network serves as an important source of professional colleagues who might provide references for jobs, advice about training opportunities, help in preparing travel scholarship applications and other forms of practical help in furthering your education or career.

The network may be 'horizontal', where all the people are peers, of similar professional status, perhaps comprising nurses only. Alternatively, the network may be 'multidimensional', with people from all levels of experience, or from a range of professional backgrounds as in the 'multi-disciplinary team'. Mauksch (1981) noted that physicians value such 'collegial' relationships with nurses as a means towards improving the overall quality of medical treatment. Professional autonomy is a doubtful concept. Interdependence, of this collegial sort, often leads to stimulation of positive developments and mutual support.

Why network?

Professional development does not end with gaining a professional qualification. Rather, this is the point where professionalism begins. The philosophies, concepts, skills and 'information technology' provided in your training were intended as the basis for a professional career. The content of any training has, of course, a short life-span. Many concepts, pieces of information and theories are superseded by new-generation theories and skills. The network will put you in touch with such new developments and help you understand them better.

Support or weaken?

Specific comments will be made later about your relationship with mentors and preceptors. Some general principles are relevant, however, to your relationships with anyone within your network. The strength of the network comes from the contributions of membership. Each member can maintain and develop the network. Equally, she can weaken the structure directly or through thoughtlessness. The following suggestions apply equally to informal and formal networks:

- Be clear about what you want and what you have to offer.
- Make it a rule always to be honest, with yourself and with others.
- Respect others in the network. This is not the same as liking them.
- Get yourself organized. Others will appreciate you getting to the point.
- Take your time. The answers you want may not be readily available, but will come with time.
- If you are given advice, consider this seriously, even if it doesn't 'feel' right at the time.
- Emphasize professional issues rather than casual chit-chat.
- Stick to any commitments made.Delivery on time will please. Early delivery will boost confidence.
- Make it clear what you can and can't do, as well as what you will or won't do.
- Keep in touch with the network, even when there is no necessary business.

Alternatively, there are some practices which are to be avoided:

- Don't pretend. Stick to what you know.
- Don't betray confidences. Loyalty and confidentiality rules.
- Don't stand back and expect to be bottle-fed. Share, listen and learn.
- Don't take offence if someone doesn't 'work' for you. Look for someone else who will.
- Don't burden everyone with all of your problems. Be selective with whom you ask to deal with what.
- Don't give concrete advice. Let others decide if your experience, or part of it, is right for them.
- Don't expect too much.

The most important ingredients of a supportive network have been shown to be 'personal respect', 'empathic attention' and 'absence of interpersonal defensiveness' (Firth *et al.*, 1986). These characteristics reflect earlier findings about the necessary conditions for interpersonal support and sharing (Truax and Carkhuff, 1967). Showing consideration for others, being aware of how they feel and having a commitment to openness and honesty, especially in emotional terms, represent the basis of a truly helpful relationship.

Any network is likely to comprise a variety of nurses, from different backgrounds, with different qualifications and status, and often with widely differing professional aspirations. Their 'use' of the network involves, in general, asking simple questions, the answers to which may have far-reaching effects. Much the same kind of questions are asked by the clinician, the educationalist, the manager or the researcher. Take the following example:

> I have this problem with Mrs Jones. Her daughter took an overdose last night and has been admitted to the psychiatric unit nearby. I don't know how to tell her. Don't know if I should tell her. I'm worried that she might start talking about her daughter. . .not knowing what has happened.

Questions:

If you were the nurse-in-charge of the psychiatric unit you might expect your colleague to telephone or visit you, to discuss the situation. I expect that your colleague would be interested to know:

> How would you tackle this situation?
> What would be your first step?
> What would you do if things went wrong? What if Mrs Jones became terribly upset?
> What are the risks involved in approaching this problem one way rather

than another, not just for Mrs Jones but for someone in similar circumstances?

How do you decide how much you are going to risk?

How do you feel about this kind of situation?

A nurse manager faced with 'personality clashes' among staff, atypical levels of absenteeism or sickness, or difficulties in implementing a quality assurance review, would probably be seeking answers to similar questions. Educationalists encountering 'difficult' students, or researchers with writer's block, face the same problem: frustration, indecision or helplessness. Having shared the problem, you show your willingness to consider the experience of others. Your colleagues in the network help you to understand your difficulties, and serve as models of 'good practice', finding answers to important questions. You may be expected to return the favour. Having identified a 'problem' and perhaps one, weak solution, members of your social network will help you to decide:

- what are the alternatives
- how they might be applied
- why the networker would employ this rather than that
- how she decides which risks to take and
- what such a situation might mean to her.

ROLE MODELS

Most of us are influenced by people with whom we have worked or enjoyed some special relationship, perhaps having 'looked up to' such people. Certainly we will have respected them for who they were and what they did. Few of us learn much from people whom we did not respect or value in some way, except perhaps how not to behave. Role models help us to develop by acting as an example which we can subsequently imitate.

Social learning: the modelling effect

Bandura (1977) described the rules and conventions of 'culturally appropriate behaviour' as 'social learning'. Social learning theory has three key components:

- People are more likely to imitate models who are prestigious, either because of strength, power or possessions.
- People are more likely to try to imitate the behaviour of models similar to themselves, than dissimilar models. In effect, people are less likely to try to imitate the performance of 'models' whose skills or knowledge is much greater than their own. Such 'masters' may be respected greatly, but may be seen as too good to try to emulate.
- People are more likely to imitate patterns of behaviour which are

'reinforced', rather than punished, i.e. actions which produce a positive outcome.

These lead to a range of possibilities for the identification of role models. Nurses in authority, perhaps reflected in special titles, uniform dress or even size of office and furnishings, may serve as a significant model to junior staff because of their rank and status. However, not everyone is 'turned on' by authority. Indeed, Bandura's work with deviant adolescents showed that authority models were unconditionally rejected by delinquents. Within nursing, a proportion of staff will not respond to the 'authority' model. A peer-role model, such as a colleague or fellow student, might be best. If the model shares similar beliefs and attitudes towards nursing this will improve her standing as a positive role model. In either case the principles and practice of the role model must 'work'. Bandura's delinquents were loathe to imitate the behaviour of conformist adolescents who were culturally alienated from them. Neither would they copy other delinquents whose behaviour resulted in conviction. The strongest authority model is one who can demonstrate effectiveness.

The good nurse

Social learning principles are supported by nursing research. Although these principles apply in most situations, where different values and standards of 'normal behaviour' apply, careful selection of the 'right' model is necessary. Although senior nurses, such as tutors and nurse-in-charge, will be influential to the learner (Kramer, 1974) colleagues are more likely to be the biggest influence as her career develops. Early in her career the novice nurse needs to see examples of how those more experienced take risks, establish positive relationships, respond to frustrations, accept responsibility, assert themselves, enjoy their work, relate to colleagues, recognize their assets and constructively criticize their deficiencies. Perhaps most of all she needs to see how she can use her self, in a creative way, and can respond to the many challenges in nursing. The model of the 'good nurse' is likely to possess leadership skill, independence, sensitivity, friendliness, helpfulness, emotional support, intelligence, thinking skills, manual skills, composure and humour (Smith, 1965). All of these serve as an incentive to imitation.

Four models

Four main kinds of role model, all offering different kinds of development, have been described. Nurse teachers are expected to demonstrate their ability to teach, as well as their general knowledge of, and competence in nursing (Rauen, 1974). In the clinical setting the 'nurse practitioner' serves as an example of positive care based upon concern, compassion and commitment, supported by appropriate theoretical knowledge and practical skills (Delaney, 1969). The clinical nurse specialist is a model for clinical development and expertise, introducing innovative practice based upon sound judgement, theoretical knowledge and flexibility (Georgopoulos and Christman, 1970). Finally, the senior nurse with overall responsibility will provide a model of leadership and management. Given her position of authority, she is in a position to reinforce staff in her charge and thereby reinforce her own status as a positive role model.

Most readers will select their own role models. Imitation of 'significant others' usually is subconscious and you might find yourself following the example of a respected colleague without being aware that you are doing so. In some situations imitation of role models might be recommended. Educationalists or managers might decide that the most appropriate way for an individual to learn or develop existing skills and knowledge, is through example. Tutors often allocate learners to specific clinical settings so that appropriate modelling can take place. Similarly, managers might decide that the easiest way for a new member of staff to complete her induction would be through 'shadowing' an experienced team member, learning the ropes through modelling.

THE PRECEPTOR

The kind of modelling noted above is limited in scope. The 'learner' can only acquire the skills or knowledge which the model is able to demonstrate. The orientation of staff to a new work setting or to changes in role function can be facilitated by a preceptor, who is a special kind of role model. Although the objective here is to help the 'preceptee' adjust to new demands, the preceptor's role is partly modelling and partly facilitative: helping the preceptee realize, or create, skills or knowledge specific to herself.

The relationship is usually very short term with a clear set of objectives and expectations. Usually selected by the nurse manager, the preceptor aims to promote the acquisition of new skills or knowledge through direct role modelling. This specific kind of helping towards increased professional development, is often called 'facilitation' (Beckett and Wall, 1985). (The concept of the preceptor is reviewed by Shamian and Inhaber (1985).) Increasingly the concept is being translated into more formal preceptor posts. Five main requirements have been identified:

1. The preceptor needs to work directly alongside the preceptee (Friesen and Conahan, 1980);
2. The preceptor's role should be clearly defined;
3. Preparation for the preceptor's role should be matched to her experience and the demands involved (Friesen and Conahan, 1980);

4. What is required of the preceptor, and the expectations of the pre-ceptee, should be clearly stated;
5. The contribution made by the preceptor should be acknowledged by the organization (McGrath and Koewing, 1978). In some cases this might involve regrading or some form of non-financial remuneration.

The preceptor should possess specific qualities which are central to the facilitation of learning. She needs to be:

- actively involved in the area which will be the focus for the preceptee;
- competent and knowledgeable about this area of care, management, research or education;
- aware of the goals of her work with the preceptee;
- able to make decisions, especially concerning the setting of priorities and time management;
- able to communicate fluently and assertively;
- interested in the professional development of nurses in general;
- willing to take constructive criticism.

Preceptee role

The preceptee should be encouraged to adopt the role of the 'learner', even where she is already highly experienced. In particular she should set the following personal objectives:

- know the goals of the contract with the preceptor;
- treat each contact with the preceptor as a learning experience;
- identify clearly the information, reasoning, skills, issues and problems presented in different situations;
- practice skills or study information as 'homework assignments';
- critically evaluate the preceptor. Give her feedback in order to help her become more aware of her own actions and to clarify your own perceptions.

Modelling stages

The preceptor's focus should not be purely upon behaviour. Initially the preceptor should clarify what needs to be done, clarifying the preceptee's present knowledge and expectations as a convenient starting point. Assuming that she knows nothing, or is not aware of what she needs to know, may waste time. Agreeing upon goals is the starting point.

At this stage it is important to establish how the preceptee feels about the task, job, or role in general. She may feel that the role is threatening, com-plex, dangerous or exciting. Alternatively, she might view the situation as boring, irrelevant, unimportant or demeaning. How she feels about what is to follow will be an important 'scene setter' for the learning situation. The preceptor now has the opportunity to discuss her own feelings, these serving as either support or a contrast.

Identification of what needs to be done and the rationale underlying a specific procedure or policy can now be presented. Talking the preceptee through the stages of a complex task, as the preceptor demonstrates, can be helpful. The aim here is to help the preceptee to know, or understand, what is required of her.

Finally, the preceptee practises imitation of her model (the preceptor). Where a complex procedure is involved, this is best done in discrete stages. Each stage is practised separately and then linked to the others in gradual progression, thereby illustrating the logical relationship or sequence.

Learning is most likely to take place if the preceptee is not unnecessarily anxious. The preceptor needs to make her 'charge' feel as comfortable as possible. Although there are likely to be some clear goals, which the preceptor might model, some flexibility may be of advantage. In some cases the preceptee may bring previous experience from a quite different area of work, which might be adapted to the new situation. Similarly, you may have thoughts on 'how' you can fulfil the role being introduced to you by the preceptor. Given these considerations the preceptor needs to establish a balance between the facilitative and modelling aspects of her role. This aim might be achieved indirectly by the preceptor avoiding the following:

- Don't 'show off' your superior knowledge. Do try to relate your experience to the needs of the preceptee.
- Don't use this relationship to boost you own self-importance. Do enjoy helping your colleague.
- Don't behave like a mother hen. Do let you colleague tell and show you what she needs or wants.
- Don't encourage dependency. Do aim to make yourself redundant as quickly as possible.
- Don't try to control. Do aim to be flexible, take turns, listen and learn yourself.
- Don't encourage gratitude. Do show how important this is to you also. Share the pleasure of learning.
- Don't take this responsibility if you don't want it. Do the preceptee a favour by trying to arrange a substitute if you feel that it is in her best interests.

THE MENTOR

A different kind of learning-through-facilitation can be arranged by a mentor. Although the concept of the mentor is relatively new in the UK, a large body of literature exists in North America (May, Meleis and Winstead-Fry, 1982; Pardue, 1983). The key distinction between a preceptor and a mentor is that whereas the former is assigned to help the nurse, the latter is selected by the nurse herself (the protégée). As the concept is introduced to Britain, the overlap between mentors and preceptors is perhaps being exaggerated at the expense of the important distinctions (Morris, John and Keen, 1988). Mentorship requires commitment, on both sides, to a relationship which may stretch over months and years, rather than weeks. Mentorship involves a sophisticated, perhaps mature, professional taking a special interest in the development of the nurse's career, and perhaps also the development of the 'whole person'. The mentor is the guide, adviser, support and sometimes friend and tutor. The nurse is her protégée. This kind of relationship has its roots in Greek mythology. Odysseus always sought the advice of an old friend before embarking on his travels: that friend being Mentor (Grahn, 1987).

The mentor has been described as a combination of a good parent, good friend, godfather, rabbi and coach (May, Meleis and Winstead-Fry, 1982). The mentor, unlike either the role model or the preceptor makes a special committment to her protégée. Mentorship is voluntary, often conducted outside work hours, and offering no financial incentive to the mentor. Mentorship aims to promote significant growth in the protégée. The mentor–protégée relationship develops only when the following criteria are present:

- The mentor possesses the professional knowledge and reputation necessary to meet your requirements.
- Both you and your mentor must share mutual respect for each others' goals and also existing accomplishments.
- The mentor needs to be able to 'open doors' for you, providing access to other professionals and situations which might aid your development.
- Your aims must match the mentor's ideals of professional development. It should not be forgotten that a nurse can have more than one mentor. Indeed, where you have a wide range of professional needs it may be unrealistic to expect any one person to be able to help you realize all of these ambitions.

Working together

Face-to-face meetings are valuable for in-depth exploration of specific issues. However, much of the 'work' may be conducted at a distance. Telephone conversations and letters can set up library assignments, mini-projects, clarify specific technical issues, review existing objectives and set new objectives. Audio-tape recordings, with prepared questions, responses or other comments, can be exchanged. The mentor–protégée relationship should reflect the needs of both parties, employing mechanisms most comfortable and convenient to both.

Finding a mentor

Your first task is to identify someone who might fulfil the requirements of a mentor. You need to know your goals before tracking the guide who might take you there. Once your plan is clear you can assess the availability of local mentors who may be educationalists, researchers, clinical specialists, or administrators. Identify those who are educationally and experientially knowledgeable in your area of interest. According to May, Meleis and Winstead-Fry (1982) the ideal mentor:

- is confident;
- posesses the personal qualities needed to form good relationships;
- has a clear self-concept;
- commands respect;
- is willing and able to give of herself;
- has a personal interest in your professional development.

Being concerned about your professional development, at whatever level, you will want someone who cares about you and your professional needs; and who can help you to realize your objectives and stimulate you towards your own professional fulfilment. Darling (1984) suggested that protégées commonly identified three specific roles which were most 'needed'. These reflected the characteristics of the effective mentor. Protégées wanted someone who could inspire them. Protégées are usually attracted to someone they respect, look up to or wish to emulate. The inspirer role also communicates an image, or professional ideal which is meaningful to the protégée and the mentor has the charisma to stimulate the protégée towards attainment of this ideal. You will also want your mentor to act as an investor, showing that she believes in you, investing in you through some direct action. Finally, you need a supporter, providing emotional encouragement and reassurance, instilling confidence and encouraging risk-taking.

If a mentor is not to be found locally contacts made at conferences, workshops and other training venues may either identify a potential mentor, or provide an introduction to someone who might consider this role. If introduction by a mutual acquaintance is not possible, a more assertive approach might be needed: a polite introduction or expression of interest in the area of the mentor's teaching, specialty or research, can be followed up later by a more direct request for support. A third alternative is to approach those who have published in your area of interest.

FORMAL GROUPS

National organizations

The broadest area of support open to you exists in a range of formal groups, societies or other organizations. All countries have organizations representing an 'official' voice for one nursing specialty or another: from the National Association of Theatre Nurses to the Mental Handicap Nurses Information Exchange. Some are sub-sections of larger organizations. In Great Britain, for example, the Royal College of Nursing (RCN), has a number of societies with interests in specific specialties, nursing education, management and research. Members of the RCN can register their interest in any number of different societies, receiving newsletters, advance notices of conferences, book lists etc.

Local organizations

Many national organizations support groups which operate at a local level. These adhere to the same principles and ideology of the main body but are more concerned to meet needs specific to their local area. The Community Psychiatric Nurses Association (CPNA) is a national organization which supports smaller regional groups who arrange training workshops and study days. Through appointed local representatives the opinion of individual members can be canvassed for onward transmission to the national executive, and local groups can play their part in shaping policy, official statements and the general philosophy of the national organization. One local group, worthy of special mention is the research interest group. This is usually not affiliated to any specific national organization, but serves as a local forum for professional development using published and ongoing research as the key stimulus.

CONCLUSION

This chapter has outlined some of the possible areas of social support which might aid your professional development. The range of possibilities is very great indeed and, as a result, four discrete (yet related) forms of support have been described. These examples might reflect the concept of 'horses-for-courses'. The kind of support needed is determined by the need itself. Nurses who are feeling demoralized by organizational changes at their place of work, might benefit from sharing these feelings with colleagues who are willing to listen and have the capability to 'empathize'. Such 'sharing' might end there or might lead to a more active response to what is seen as a personal professional problem. You might feel that such a casual, or informal, network does not meet your specific needs, and turn to a more organized forum, at local or national level, for support. In either case, knowing what is your need, is the key to finding the right kind of support.

Role models represent a more specific kind of support. Nurses wishing to extend themselves can learn much from 'unofficial' learning from a model who reflects the skills, ideals or knowledge which is relevant to them. Nurse managers are increasingly recognizing the need to arrange such modelling or facilitation of learning on a more official basis, the preceptor being an example of such 'conducted' learning in practice. Finally, if you wish to set your own professional goals, and aim to embark on a longer-term course of professional goals, and aim to embark on a longer-term course of professional development, the mentor–protégée relationship seems most appropriate.

REFERENCES

Bandura, A. (1977) *Social Learning Theory*, Prentice-Hall, New Jersey.

Beckett, C. and Wall, M. (1985) Role of the clinical facilitator. *Nurse Education Today*, **5**(6), 259–62.

Darling, L.A.W. (1984) What do nurses want in a mentor? *Journal of Nursing Administration*, **14**(10), 42–4.

Delaney, P.E. (1969) Selecting learning experiences which encourage deviant behaviour. *American Journal of Nursing*, **69**(4), 800–3.

Durkheim, E. (1933) *The Division of Labour in Society*, Macmillan, London.

Firth, H., McIntee, J., McKeown, P. and Britton P. (1986) Interpersonal support among nurses at work. *Journal Advanced Nursing*, **11**(3), 273–82.

Friesen, L. and Conahan, B.J. (1980) Clinical preceptor program: strategy for new graduate orientation. *Journal of Nursing Administration*, **10**(4), 18–23.

Georgopoulos, B.S. and Christman, L. (1970) The clinical nurse specialist: A role model. *American Journal of Nursing*, **70**(5), 1030–9.

Grahn, G. (1987) Preceptorships and mentors. *Cancer Nursing*, **10**(1), 181–5.

Kramer, M. (1974) *Reality Shock: Why nurses leave nursing*, Mosby, St Louis.

McGrath, B.J. and Koewing, J.R. (1978) A clinical preceptorship for new graduate nurses. *Journal of Nursing Administration*, **8**(10), 12–8.

Mauksch, I.G. (1981) Nurse-physician collaboration: A changing relationship. *Journal of Nursing Administration*, **11**(5), 35–8.

May, K., Meleis, A.I. and Winstead-Fry, P. (1982) Mentorship for scholarliness: Opportunies and dilemmas. *Nursing Outlook*, **30**(1), 22–8.

Morris, N., John, G. and Keen, T. (1988) Mentors: Learning the ropes. *Nursing Times and Nursing Mirror*, **84**(46), 24–7.

Pardue, S. (1983) The who-what-why of mentor teacher/graduate student relationship. *Journal of Nursing Education*, **22**(1), 32–7.

Rauen, K.C. (1974) The clinical instructor as the model. *Journal of Nursing Education*, **13**(3), 33–9.

Shamian, J. and Inhaber, R. (1985) The concept and practice of preceptorship in contemporary nursing: A review of pertinent literature. *International Journal of Nursing Studies*, **22**(2), 79–88.

Smith, K.M. (1965) Discrepancies in the role of specific values of head nurses and nursing education. *Nursing Research*, **14**(3), 196–202.

Truax, B.B. and Carkhuff, R.R. (1967) *Towards Effective Counselling and Psychotherapy*, Aldine, New York.

Chapter 21

Collective assertiveness

DESMOND CORMACK

Chapter 3 focused on individual assertiveness. However, there are many circumstances in which you, if acting in isolation from others, can have relatively little impact. Examples include influencing nationally agreed arrangements for pay and conditions of service, influencing the content of nurse education programmes, and influencing government expenditure on the National Health Service. Similarly, a number of local issues can be best addressed as a result of collective (as opposed to individual) assertiveness. Examples include rearrangement of existing nursing staff shifts, provision of transport for community nurses, planning for movement of mentally ill/mentally handicapped patients from hospital to the community, and the availability of resources for continuing education.

It is not being suggested that individual and collective assertiveness exist in isolation from each other. Indeed, it might be argued that collective assertiveness is an amalgam of, and results from, the extent to which assertiveness does/does not exist in the individuals who make up the group. Nurses, in common with other work groups, have long recognized that some issues can be best addressed on a collective, rather than an individual, basis. For the most part, these issues are ones which affect groups of staff or, in many instances, the entire work force. Some may be unidisciplinary or, in the case of health service financing, affect all of those who provide and receive health care.

There has been considerable recent debate on the extent to which nursing as a profession demonstrates its collective assertiveness. Styles (1987) in a discussion of the future of nursing wrote:

> We turn against ourselves. A self-ravaging autoimmune disease rages. We present ourselves divided, in disarray, and less powerful in the public arena. The downward spiral to our demise begins. Economic leverage is lost. A profession of not only potential but actual importance is diminished.... My wish for the future then, is that we may realize that we must free and aid nursing to rise to its destiny. We must work together to possess those tools of progress: expert knowledge, public sanction to use that expertise, and power in the political processes.

Kay (1988) referred to the endemic low self-esteem which pervades nursing. Griffiths (1987) suggested that: 'One of the problems with the nursing profession is a bit of an inferiority complex as to their real capabilities. They had lived so long in the shadows of the doctors that they weren't really seeing what the potential was for them.' This abrogation of power in favour of medical staff has also been referred to by Robinson and Strong (1988).

There is clearly cause for concern regarding the ability of the nursing profession to exercise collective assertiveness. This concern does not wholly result from a recognition of the need for nurses generally to exercise political power for solely selfish ends. Although one important aspect of exercising such power is to ensure that the nursing profession, and individuals within it, are properly rewarded, many of the issues relate to the quality of care, and resources available, for patients. One important means of achieving these aims is for nurses to work together and collectively influence those who are in a position to make the final decisions regarding these issues. Collective assertiveness can be exercised in the workplace, via nursing leadership, political power, trade unions and professional organizations, and by influencing the work of nursing's statutory bodies.

THE WORKPLACE

Many nurses work in institutions, or in peripheral units which are associated with a parent hospital. Others such as community nurses may work in *relative* isolation from colleagues; however, all will invariably be part of a larger local, district or area work force. Thus, most nurses are part of a professional group who share the same aims. Invariably, a range of issues arise in relation to a workforce in which there is some agreement with regard to the desirable outcome of addressing these issues. In these circumstances, it is necessary for the individuals concerned to meet, discuss these issues, and develop a common view with regard to them. Discussion of the issues may frequently, although not necessarily always, be confined to a nursing group. On other occasions, the issue may be of a multi-disciplinary type which requires input from other disciplines. In either event, it is essential that a collective assertive approach be used to make the views of the nursing staff group known to those who can influence the issue being discussed. For example, a nursing staff group would be perfectly entitled (indeed obliged) to make known its views concerning any topic which affected that group. Similarly, if an issue related to only part of a workforce it might be appropriate for that part to seek the support of the entire workforce. Frequently, the collective view of the nursing staff might be made known to such groups as medical colleagues, hospital administrators, the nursing management system, or to some external body. The platforms for the presentation and prior formulation of such views might be an ad hoc group formed specifically for this purpose or, alternatively, by one or more of the professional organizations/trade unions who represent nursing staff in this particular work place.

What is being suggested here is that there are many 'local' issues which can be best resolved via collective, rather than individual, assertiveness. If the machinery for making such collective representation does not already exist in a particular workplace, it is essential that those involved construct such a forum. Ideally, this is an ongoing process in which a structure is created whereby nurses (collectively) can make representation to and influence other individuals, groups and organizations. Cavanaugh (1985) referred to this collective approach as 'building a coalition'. She wrote:

> Building a coalition is the most visible way of working with someone else's self-interest. Together each of you can achieve a goal that separately was out of your reach. Coalitions can be formed by people with the same goal, but they can only be formed by people who have different (although not opposing) goals and they are willing to support one another in each of their quests.

That writer also discussed the development of strategies as a means of achieving collective goals. She wrote:

> Strategy is the diagnosis, planning and execution of an effective campaign to achieve a well-thought-out, purposeful goal. It is based on politics, not logic or rationality (although both are part of a good strategy). . . . Strategy means recognizing that everyone has self-interests in every situation, and working with those self-interests to achieve your goal.

The achievement of goals which have been identified by the nursing staff group need not necessarily be in conflict with the overall goal of the organization. Indeed, if such conflict does exist then one has to question whether the goal is appropriate or reasonable.

LEADERSHIP

The expression of collective assertiveness is frequently only made possible by the ability and willingness of an individual to take over a leadership role. This role may relate to all or some of the following; identification of the issue, organizing collective discussion of the issue, recording and summarizing the outcome of that discussion and presentation of the outcome to other individuals and/or organizations. Such a representation may be in a verbal and/or written form.

For some time, nursing has relied on leaders who held that position by virtue of their place in an authoritative and hierarchical nursing structure. Some such 'leaders' may have lacked the authority and assertiveness which was required to express the views of nursing staff and ensure that these views were taken into account. This criticism of nursing leadership, although changing, was applicable to part of the spectrum of nursing leadership from local to national level. With regard to the national leadership of nursing, particularly as it relates to the leadership of professional organizations, *Nursing Times* (1986) stated that 'the days have gone when nurse leaders could be quiet administrators or decorative figureheads.' Nurses are now more critical of the skills of those in leadership positions, and make increased (although reasonable) demands on those who lead them.

In terms of national leadership, and in relation to those leaders who hold positions of authority in the nursing hierarchy, there is little that can be done with regard to effecting immediate change if these individuals do not function well. However, many nurses have an informal leadership role within local staff groups. Nurses are becoming much more discerning in terms of identifying such individuals and assisting them in representing (leading) nurses on an informal basis. This is particularly so of nursing in the work place, and in presenting those collective views which are local as opposed to national. These individuals enable us to exercise political power, which is the capacity to achieve change.

POLITICAL POWER

Politics may be defined as any activity concerned with the acquisition of power. Power may be defined as the ability or capacity to achieve change. Thus, political power may be defined as any activity concerned with the acquisition of the means of achieving change. Until recently, nurses have not been perceived as being 'political animals'. The perception of nurses has traditionally been as subservient, reacting to, rather than causing, change, and lacking in the individual and collective assertiveness which are prerequisites to the acquisition of political power. During the past two decades this position has gradually changed to one in which individuals and groups are more forcefully exercising political power in relation to a number of aspects of nursing.

Nursing, in order to remain a profession, and further develop its professionalism, is recognizing the need to enter the 'political arena'. Professional groups with a coherent knowledge and power base tend to have the greatest impact on those who make decisions relating to nursing collectively. Nursing undoubtedly has the power base which is necessary for enabling it to contribute to all aspects of decision-making. Indeed, in relation to nursing, nurses are the only group who have the expertise which must be the basis of such a contribution. At national level there exists a number of professional organizations/trade unions which enable individual nurses to exercise professional power. Unfortunately, a relatively small number of nurses belong to these organizations; additionally, the nursing power base is considerably diluted by virtue of there being a number of such organizations. This topic will be discussed later in this chapter.

Exercising political power in the work place is dependent on the formulation of coherent and collective strategies. Such strategies can only be formulated if the groups concerned meet to discuss the relevant issues. In some outdated management systems, such an approach may be perceived as being a threat to those in authority. Other (more enlightened) managers welcome this opportunity which will enable groups of nurses to formulate and present coherent and well-thought-out collective views. Frequently, senior nurses meet on a regular basis to discuss issues of common interest, as do general managers. It seems reasonable and appropriate that nurses at other levels (for example, ward sisters/charge nurses) within a defined area of functioning should also meet to discuss issue of common interest. Increasingly, there is becoming normal practice.

Contemporary nurses, to be effective and successful, must have an expertise which extends beyond planning, delivering and controlling clinical care, and other managerial, teaching or research functions. By the time a nurse reaches a particular level of status or experience, success and failure criteria are extended to include personal assertiveness and authority, exercising political power, and functioning within a particular ethos and style of an organization. As with career development generally, that which a nurse receives from and gives to an organization is optimized by exercising political power.

Exercising political power on a collective basis is facilitated by:

- Identifying and collaborating with others who are concerned regarding a particular issue and who are able to formulate shared strategies for addressing that issue.
- Establishing alliances with others, who are not directly involved in the issue, who are in a position to influence the outcome of required change.
- Using all possible channels of communication in order to achieve change. To some extent, nurses are inhibited in that there is an expectation that they will confine any 'politicing' to their immediate superiors in the nursing hierarchy. Fortunately, this desire of nurses 'in authority' to control the activity of others is diminishing. However, there is sufficient desire for control on the part of a minority of senior nurses to warrant the injection of a word of caution. Becoming involved in power politics is potentially damaging to those involved, particularly those who are seen to take a leadership role. It is essential, therefore, to create, and work within, a climate where this form of activity is regarded as the norm.

- Knowing how decisions are made increases the chance of success. To believe that proposals for change stand on their own merit is naïve. A range of politically motivated factors inevitably influence proposals for change, particularly if these proposals affect other individuals or groups, or if the proposals have resource implications.
- Establishing priorities for change is essential. All proposals must be seen in the context of a range of others which compete for resources and for the attention of those who are in a position to effect change. Additionally, a proposal might have a number of discrete (although inter-related) elements which may offer the opportunity for the implementation of partial change.
- Being willing to compromise is a possibility which should always be borne in mind. In short, partial success is better than none. Although there should be no compromise in issues which are ethically or morally founded, maintaining a position of flexibility and manoeuvrability will make success more possible.
- Identifying major issues as (opposed to those which are relatively unimportant) will enable the focus to be maintained on those which are important. Major issues which are contaminated by a number of trivial ones are difficult to discuss and present in a meaningful way.
- Being politically aware enables the issues to be presented in the most appropriate way, at the best possible time, and to those parts of the organization which are most likely to be in agreement. Although deception is not being recommended, it is necessary to use strategies with maximum effect.

TRADE UNIONS/PROFESSIONAL ORGANIZATIONS

In virtually all countries which have a well-developed nursing profession in which nurses are required to be registered/licenced, the option to become a member of a trade union/professional organization is available. In many countries nurses have access to membership of a range of organizations. Some organizations have, traditionally, a function which is primarily that of a trade union. Other organizations have a role which emcompasses both trade union and professional activities. Although there is considerable blurring between the major functions of these two types of organizations, there remains a strong perception of there being considerable differences between the two. Clay (1987) the then General Secretary of the Royal College of Nursing (RCN), described that organization as a 'professional' trade union. In addition to having a range of functions which relate to the 'pay and conditions' of its membership, the RCN is involved in, and addresses, a range of professional and educational issues relating to nursing. Clay described these activities as being in addition to the trade union activities of the RCN. He described these as consuming as much, if not more, of the time of the RCN. Thus, some organizations such as the RCN combine a trade union and professional range of activities. Other organizations such as the Confederation of Health Service Employees (COHSE) have traditionally been perceived as focusing mainly, if not exclusively, on trade union activities in which they address issues relating to the pay and conditions of the nursing work force. Virtually all organizations which represent nurses are becoming increasingly involved in the 'professional' aspect of their functioning. Delamothe (1988) described the Confederation of Health Service Employees (COHSE) as follows:

> COHSE resulted from the amalgamation in 1946 of the National Asylum Worker's Union and the Poor Law Worker's Trade Union. Its members came from all part of the health service: two-thirds of its 220 000 members are nurses. COHSE's heartlands were the large psychiatric hospitals, many of which are closing. Recently COHSE has become much more active in community care.

Of the 146 000 'nurses' who are members of COHSE, Delamothe (1988) gives the breakdown as follows:

> Trained nurses (including midwives): 60%
> Nurses in training: 16%
> Unqualified (assistant) staff, those who are neither trained nor in training; 24%

Thus, COHSE, which has a membership of 220 000 (74 000 of whom are not nurses) has a nurse/nursing assistant membership of which approximately one-quarter are unqualified, the remaining three-quarters being either trained or in training.

Unlike the Confederation of Health Service Employees which is typical of many trade unions to which nurses belong, the Royal College of Nursing has a membership which is presently composed exclusively of qualified nurses, and of nurses in training. Delamothe (1988) described the Royal College of Nursing as being:

> Founded in 1916 (as the College of Nursing) the RCN with 265 000 members is now the ninth largest union in Britain and the fastest growing. In recent years the RCN has become much more 'political'. In 1960 it finally admitted men to its ranks: they now comprise 7.4% of its membership, and men hold four of its top five administrative positions. Membership was extended to student nurses in 1968 and to enrolled and pupil nurses in 1970. Nursing auxilliaries may not join.

The main objectives of the Royal College of Nursing as set out in its Royal Charter include:

To promote the science and art of nursing and the better education and training of nurses.... To promote the advance of nursing as a profession.... To promote the professional standing and interests of members of the nursing profession.... To assist nurses who, by reason of adversity, ill health or otherwise, are in need of assistance of any nature.... (Royal College of Nursing 1988, p. 5)

It might be argued that the real political power of which nursing is capable of achieving can only be realized if nurses are active members of a trade union/professional organization. More particularly, it might be argued that this power can only be fully realized if nurses are members of a single organization which is specific to nursing. The reality is that many nurses are not members of any such organizations (a conservative estimate would be that approximately 65% of nurses are members of any organization). Many nurses who are members of an organization belong to one which represents nursing and disciplines other than nursing. Finally it is probable that the majority of nurses are passive members of the organization to which they belong. The fact that nursing in the UK is represented by a number of professional/trade union organizations seriously compromises the political assertiveness of the nursing profession. The organizations which currently represent nurses in the UK include:

Association of Nurse Administrators
Association of Supervisors of Midwives
Confederation of Health Service Employees
Health Visitor's Association
Managerial, Administrative, Technical and Supervisory Association
National and Local Government Officers' Association
National Union of Public Employees
Royal College of Midwives
Royal College of Nursing
Scottish Association of Nurse Administrators
Scottish Health Visitors' Association

In the foreseeable future it is highly probable that this position of disunity will continue to exist, indeed it is likely to be sustained by the variety of organizations which represent nurses (all of whom claim to be providing the best service for our profession). However, it is possible that, in the long term, a single organization will emerge which will represent the views of the vast majority of nurses, and enable the profession to fully exercise its political power. There is growing evidence to suggest that individuals within many of the existing organizations see this as a necessary development, and are placing the issue on the professional agenda. Cole (1987) referred to the deep differences which existed between the Royal College of Nursing and two other trade unions, the Confederation of Health Service Employees and the National Union of Public Employees.

On occasions these differences have emerged as a result of the organizations using different means of achieving the same end. Turner (1988) wrote: 'Relations between the RCN and other trade unions representing nurses have never been cordial. But in recent months matters have become severely strained as the organizations' different approaches have been highlighted by a series of health protests.' Similar references to inter-union conflict were discussed by Jane (1988).

There is a widely-held view that all nurses should hold membership of an organization which represents them at national level. My own view on this issue is uncompromising; it is that all professional nurses should belong to a union/professional organization, and that they use that membership to influence its work. The least that an individual nurse will obtain from such membership is to be given advice/legal assistance/insurance protection in times of adversity. Quite correctly, employers protect their interests by making use of a variety of procedures and organizations which are designed for that purpose. Employers do terminate contracts, dismiss staff, give verbal/written warnings and take other sanctions. Similarly, you have access to, and should make use of, appropriate union/professional organization support systems which will protect your interests and provide representation should this be necessary.

There is continued debate regarding the role of traditional trade unions and of organizations which have a trade union/professional function. Some writers have questioned the ability of a single organization such as the Royal College of Nursing, to combine professional and trade union/political activities (Atkinson, 1983). One important issue accompanying membership of any organization is that of withdrawing labour. During recent years nurses have become increasingly involved in strikes, and in discussions relating to whether or not this is a legitimate activity (Bolger, 1988; Vousden, 1988). These discussions have, to a large extent, highlighted the potential conflict between belonging to a profession, and membership of a trade union/professional organization. Beletz (1983) concluded that: 'Until nurses develop solidarity and a commitment to the maximization of their bargaining power, the use of the strike and picketing by nurses will be of dubious effectiveness.' Baumgart (1983) in a discussion of the conflicting demands of professionalism and unionism, discussed the complimentary, although differing roles of the professional organizations and trade unions Kristensen (1987) suggested that professional interests were inadequately met in coalitions between trade unions and professional organizations.

Whatever the outcome of the power struggles between trade unions and professional organizations, and of those bodies which attempt to serve both functions, there can be little doubt that there is need for such organizations to continue to represent the interests of nurses, and for every nurse to be a member of such a body. The International Council of Nurses (1987) commented that studies have consistently proven that workers covered by collective aggreements had better terms and conditions of employment than those who did not. The goal for the future must be to protect and improve the working conditions of nurses, and to ensure the development of nursing as a profession. See Holleran (1989) for a description of the role of International Council Of Nurses and the contribution of that organization to 'The politics of nursing'.

STATUTORY BODIES

In most, but by no means all, countries there exists a statutory body which is responsible for the education of nurses, for the registering of all trained nurses, and for ensuring that registered nurses conform to an agreed code of professional conduct. In some areas such as the UK, such a body functions at a national level; in others such as the USA this responsibility lies within each of the states. In the UK, the United Kingdom Central Council for Nursing, Midwifery and Health Visiting (UKCC) is charged with the responsibility for ensuring and maintaining the quantity and quality of nurse education, for approving the areas in which nurses will be trained, maintaining standards regarding the examination of nurses in training, and for ensuring compliance with our code of professional conduct.

The UKCC consists of 45 members: 7 from each of the National Boards, and 17 members appointed by the Secretary of State. Each of the four countries which form the UK have a National Board which is composed of;

The English National Board for Nursing, Midwifery and Health Visiting has 45 members: 20 elected nurses, 5 elected midwives, 5 elected health visitors, and 15 members who are appointed by government ministers.

The National Board for Nursing, Midwifery and Health Visiting for Scotland has 36 members: 16 elected nurses, 4 elected midwives, 4 elected health visitors, and 12 members appointed by government ministers.

The National Board for Nursing, Midwifery and Health Visiting for Northern Ireland has 35 members: 4 elected health visitors, 4 elected midwives, 16 elected nurses, and 11 members appointed by government ministers.

The Welsh National Board for Nursing, Midwifery and Health Visiting has 35 members: 4 elected health visitors, 4 elected midwives, 16 elected nurses, and 11 members appointed by government ministers.

Clearly, each of the National Boards, and the Central Council, have a heavy representation of elected nurses, midwives and health visitors. These elected members constitute an important means by which nurses can individually, and collectively, influence the status, future direction of, and development of the nursing profession. It is now normal practice for individuals who seek election to these bodies to make public statements regarding the contribution which they feel they can make, special areas of interest, and the issues which they feel should be addressed. In so doing, they give 'rank and file' staff the opportunity to support candidates who have views similar to their own, or who have the ability to generally influence the direction and development of the nursing profession. Similarly, the 'high visibility' of nurses, midwives and health visitors who are elected to these bodies provide the opportunity for individuals or groups to make their views known to the National Boards and to the Central Council via these individuals. In short, by voting for particular individuals, and maintaining an input through them to the various bodies, it is possible to exercise power and influence opinion.

Exercising individual and collective assertiveness via the National Boards and Central Council is dependent on developing and maintaining an involvement in the work of these bodies. There is, however, some evidence to suggest that individual nurses are playing a less then assertive part, particularly in relation to the election of members of the National Boards. Cole (1988) cites Colin Ralph, the UKCC's registrar and chief executive as saying in relation to forthcoming elections: 'The next five years will cover a period of unprecedented change and challenge for the profession. It is imperative that nurses, midwives and health visitors play their rightful part in these elections. By doing so they will not only be helping to regulate their profession but to shape it future.' In the event, approximately one-quarter of those elegible to do so, cast their vote. Clearly, there is an obvious need to be concerned about the relatively low number of nurses, midwives and health visitors who take the opportunity to select those who will lead the profession.

The UKCC and the four National Boards provide a framework for developing nursing, midwifery and health visiting on a nationwide basis. As with all legitimate avenues for exercising collective and individual assertiveness, we all have full opportunity to influence the profession via the statutory bodies.

Unity is indeed strength. It can, and should, be the means by which we collectively and individually influence the present and future direction of nursing practice, management, education and research. In a wider context, it also is the means by which we influence other health care professionals, government and, most importantly, society.

REFERENCES

Atkinson, B. (1983) Is the RCN too political? *Nursing Times*, **83**(42), 40.
Baumgart, A. (1983) The conflicting demands of professionalism and unionism. *International Nursing Review*, **30**(5), 150–5.
Beletz, E. (1983) Nurses' commitment to militance in collective bargaining.

International Nursing Review, **30**(4), 110–7.

Bolger, T. (1988) Power and the glory. *Nursing Times*, **84**(12), 27.

Cavanaugh, D. (1985) Gamesmanship: The art of Strategizing. *Journal of Nursing Administration*, **15**(4), 38–41.

Clay, T. (1987) Professional trade unionism. *Lampada*, **12**, 34–5.

Cole, A. (1988) Your chance to pull the strings. *Nursing Times*, **84**(19), 16–8.

Cole, A. (1987) Part of the union? *Nursing Times*, **83**(44), 19.

Delamothe, T. (1988) Nursing grievances 1: Voting with their feet. *British Medical Journal*, **296**, 25–8.

Griffiths, R. (1987) News focus. The sky's the limit. *Nursing Times*, **83**(32), 16–8.

Holleran, C. (1989) The politics of nursing. *Nursing Standard*, **19**(3), 19–21.

International Council of Nurses (1987) Settlement of labour disputes. *International Nursing Review*, **34**(1), 7–8.

Jane, E. (1988) A warning on industrial action: Only a co-ordinated, national approach will succeed (letter). *Nursing Times*, **84**(8), 12.

Kay, E. (1988) Finding the manager behind the mask. *Nursing Times*, **84**(23), 40–1.

Kristensen, P. (1987) The Norwegian Nurses Association (N.S.F.) — Goals and Progress. *International Nursing Review*, **34**(1), 9–11.

Nursing Times (1986) Editorial. *Nursing Times*, **82**(47), 3.

Robinson, J. and Strong, P. (1988) *New model management: Griffiths and the N.H.S.*, University of Warwick Policy Studies Centre.

Royal College of Nursing (1988) *Members Handbook*. Royal College of Nursing, London.

Styles, M. (1987) The tarnished opportunity. *Nursing Outlook*, **35**(5), 229.

Turner, T. (1988) The divided unions. *Nursing Times*, **84**(10), 19.

Vousden, M. (1988) What the papers said. *Nursing Times*, **84**(7), 18.

Chapter 22

Preparing to leave nursing

ROBERT COOPER

THE NATURE OF NURSING EMPLOYMENT

A long unbroken career in nursing does not appear to be a reality for large numbers of female nurses employed within the National Health Service and when you consider that the Scottish Health Service Statistics (Common Services Agency, 1988) indicate that over 90% of all nurses in the service are female, the phenomenon of career breaks must exert a significant effect on both the individual nurse and the service in general.

Work carried out by Mackay (1988) indicated that: 'Women rarely have uninterrupted full-time careers, 50% of the leavers and 38% of the stayers in our sample had had one or more breaks from nursing.'

The occurrence of breaks suggested by Mackay's findings indicate that leaving and re-entering nursing is extremely common, and it could be naïvely assumed to cause few problems for either the individual or the service. This does not appear to be the case and it is tempting to suggest that leaving nursing, on a temporary basis, may potentially deprofessionalize the nurse. Evidence suggests that once a break in service occurs, the re-entry process is often difficult. Indeed nursing management, in some instances, has appeared to disregard the professional and personal issues surrounding re-entry and have merely seen the question as one of adequate ward cover. Additionally, many nurses who re-enter are married and have to negotiate part-time contracts. This can result in them receiving a status that can be quite different from the one they surrendered on leaving full-time employment.

According to Green (1988): 'Nursing is still seen by many as a full-time job mainly for single women. Married women who work part-time are less likely to be considered for more senior posts or for professional development and are more likely to be given more menial unskilled tasks.'

Should this be the case, then the situation is likely to be affecting around one-third of qualified nurses in the hospital service alone. The Scottish Health Service Statistics (Common Services Agency, 1988) reveal that 35.28% of qualified nursing staff are in the part-time category, and one would assume that this is a situation which might be similar to that in the other countries of the UK, and elsewhere.

Now that approaches to nursing care show evidence of changing due to an increase of interest in the notion of holistic care and the seeking of relevant theories and models on which to base nursing practice, the consequences for those seeking to re-enter nursing are more challenging. Thus, it is imperative that nurses who leave temporarily make efforts to maintain professional competence. It is against this background that many nurses have to make career choices, such choices being complicated by the fact that many nurses will leave and re-enter on more than one occasion.

Such is the present situation that work done by Waite (1988) revealed that: 'of all those (nurses) who are outside (nursing) only 50% say they expect to return.' Just how much this latter finding is a result of the prevailing conditions within nursing is difficult to judge, but it may indicate that the question of re-entry needs to be seriously addressed.

Under present circumstances nurses who leave nursing for any length of time run the risk of becoming isolated and begin to lose confidence in their nursing ability. No doubt these negative feelings begin to increase with time. Why these nurses feel this way may be related to how they were trained, educated and socialized into nursing. Authority–obedience systems, like nursing (although changing), do not generally foster professional independence and innovative thinking, thus some of the re-entry problems may lie in the culture of the nursing service and the relatively passive and subordinate attitudes such a culture appears to engender in nurses.

Attempts are being made by some health boards and authorities to overcome re-entry problems by organizing back to nursing courses, but there is no national co-ordination. More often than not such courses are a local response to an acute staff shortage and, should this short-term staffing problem be solved by this venture, then the course may be discontinued.

However, it is at least a move in the right direction to preparing out of practice nurses to assume a nursing role again. As to the success or otherwise of such courses the picture is a confusing one. Green (1988) found when evaluating back to nursing courses: '...the feeling of obsolescence was increased rather than decreased as the students became aware of how much had changed since they last nursed.' However, a contrary view was stated by Donn and Smits (1988) when it was indicated: 'The most frequent comment in the course members' evaluations was that the course had given them the confidence to return to work.'

Whether the foregoing, apparently contradictory, findings were due to course relevance, organization or teaching/learning effectiveness is difficult to say, but they may further indicate that much work has yet to be done on the subject of preparation for re-entry to nursing.

If these comments on the nature of nursing employment are valid, it must be asked if nurses, who are considering a break in their career, or are at present on one, need adopt such a seemingly passive role in relation to their professional status? There should be no reason for you to feel that because you have temporarily stepped out of the nursing role you no longer belong, or that nursing knowledge and interest be suspended until you attempt to re-enter the profession.

Nursing takes its members through to retirement, and this too can be considered a break, although a permanent one. This break needs to be considered by both you and your employer as increasing longevity and accompanying improvements in standards of health, linked with society's changing views on what old age means, makes the retirement phase of your life an extremely important one. Whether or not the nursing profession adequately assists its more mature members to prepare for this final break is open to question, it may depend more on local health board or authority's policies, than on a generally agreed national policy.

Like the advent of a temporary break, the permanent break of retirement also requires you to be active in considering what plans should be made, how such planning should be organized and when such planning should commence.

The remainder of this chapter will offer some guidance and advice to you when you are considering a career break as part of your normal life plans, or are approaching the permanent break of retirement.

TEMPORARY LEAVERS

Many nurses can be described as temporary leavers and the reasons for this leaving can be many and varied. Therefore it is worthwhile to think seriously about how you can look after your professional interests whilst out of practice.

Career development

This is an aspect of your working life which you should be thinking about even although you do not envisage a break in your career. This has become more important with the introduction of the grading system whereby you have to meet specific criteria when applying for posts. When you consider the post of staff nurse has three different gradings then it becomes obvious that relying only on basic training when applying for a post will place you at a disadvantage.

Having left nursing with the expectation of returning at some later date, consider arrangements whereby you can keep up to date with professional matters and knowledge. You may feel such a statement obvious, but experience informs us that out of practice nurses have difficulty in making positive attempts to remain informed about their profession. This keeping up to date could be particularly important if you are a nurse who is taking a break shortly after completion of basic training. At this stage you are relatively inexperienced in the art of nursing, both in the practical sense and in your working knowledge base. Just what can and should be done to keep up to date will no doubt vary from one individual to another and will obviously depend on particular circumstances.

I am frequently asked to assist nurses, who are not currently practising, to choose appropriate distance learning programmes that will help them get back into reading and study habits. This indicates that some nurses do not do much in the way of updating during their time out.

Reading

Reading about nursing is one way in which you can remain in touch, decide what to read and how often. Subscribing to a weekly journal will help you keep abreast of the major issues affecting nursing. However, such journals may be limited in their ability to keep you in touch with your own special area of nursing, and you would benefit from having access to general nursing literature. If you have any problems regarding access, contact a local college or school of nursing and negotiate with the librarian access to journals and nursing books. Even if you are some distance from such a centre a letter or phone call could initiate a potentially fruitful relationship.

Such action will require you to take the initiative for your own continuing development, but if this is tackled in a professional manner, access to such library facilities will almost certainly be made available.

How often you read is a personal matter, but it may be an advantage to establish a pattern of regular reading, even if this is only a modest hour per week. Sticking to this programme of reading would ensure 52 hours of reading in a year and this can cover a fair amount of material. When reading try not to see this as some kind of activity unrelated to actual nursing. Such reading should lead you to eventually become a more skilful nurse. There is a great danger in perceiving nursing as being composed of two separate parts, the part which is read about and the part which is done, and believing one part has little to do with the other. Indeed, work done by Melia (1987) clearly shows this to be the case amongst student nurses and one speculates as to whether this may be a reason why reading about nursing does not find a great deal of favour amongst nurses who are on breaks. Even in the absence of the opportunity to practise nursing, reading and thinking about it will improve your knowledge base, thus when the time comes to practise again it will be against a more informed background (Chapter 10).

Support groups

As an out of practice nurse you may well have opportunities to maintain occasional contacts with working colleagues, such contacts could be used to discuss present working practices. Further to this you may be able to locate other colleagues in similar circumstances to yourself and form a support group. A result of this could be that members can share the issues and seek solutions to mutual problems. Formation of a support group could lead to contact with local colleges or schools of nursing. Such a link could allow the group to negotiate monthly meetings on the premises at suitably convenient times to all concerned. Speakers could be invited from the experienced nursing staff working in the area, the subjects presented could be many and varied.

On an individual basis, or as a result of support group activity, it may be possible to participate in basic nurse training programmes, particularly now that many are based on a modular system. In my own experience, out of practice nurses have occasionally requested to sit in on specific parts of the basic training programme. For example, nurses who have medical nursing as their area of interest have approached the module teachers and have subsequently participated in the in-college part of the module. When this has occurred the participating nurses have been extremely positive in their comments. There is also an increasing demand on college services by the qualified nursing staff wishing to continue their education beyond the basic level.

Conferences and study days

To attending conferences and study days is a useful way for you to gain up date knowledge and information on your area of nursing interest. There is also the advantage of being able to talk with practising nurses, indeed some conferences have group workshops where you can become involved in discussion and debate on current nursing topics, rather than just sitting passively through a series of lectures. However, workshop activity would require one to be reasonably knowledgeable about one's craft to make a contribution. Some out of practice nurses would feel more comfortable than others in this situation, but it is an option. You must never feel that such conferences and study days are not for you just because you are on a career break, you are a qualified nurse and have a professional right to attend if the invitation is open (Chapter 13).

Voluntary work

If you can spare the time, but are not yet ready to assume full nursing responsibility, the question of voluntary work may hold some attraction for you. This can often be arranged at a local hospital or with the community services, by contacting the nurse manager. However, you must realize that it would be highly unlikely that you would be asked to function as a qualified nurse as the question of employee status and liability will arise. Nevertheless you would at least be in the nursing environment and interacting at some level with patients and nurses.

Distance learning

An increasingly popular option in continuing education for registered nurses is the distance learning method. This is usually based on units of learning materials which nurses study largely in their own time and to some extent, at their own pace. Studying usually occurs at home and is linked with group tutorials held in local colleges or schools of nursing. Nurses undertaking such studies also have a personal tutor/counsellor with whom they can make contact by letter, phone or personal visit.

I am involved with a small group of nurses who are on a career break and are using the distance learning method. They are doing this with a view to making application for a place in a back-to-nursing course. If they can show evidence of having commenced to update their nursing knowledge, on their own initiative, their chances of being selected into such courses will be enhanced as the experience of distance learning would hopefully help the nurses to feel more confident when talking about nursing at interview. The nurses I am referring to above were taken on by me after the Manpower Services Commission (now the Training Agency) negotiated on the nurses behalf. I then became the nurses contact tutor and gave advice and guidance to them during the time they are studying. As these nurses are out of work the Training Agency can offer a little financial assistance in the purchase of the learning units.

Return to nursing courses

Such courses have a number of names including, re-entry courses, back-to-nursing courses, return-to-practice courses and so on. The indications are that they can be very useful to the participants. Some courses have a system of protected practice whereby the returning nurse is allocated a mentor who 'shadows' her during the clinical experience part of the course. Donn and Smits (1988) found when investigating such a course that 'The protected practice was valued by all participants...' and one could see that this could give the returning nurse the confidence to take up the challenge of nursing once more.

These courses sometimes have to be paid for by the participants and others are free. The question of charging lies entirely with those who organize such courses and one hears of figures of between fifty and a hundred pounds being charged for a course lasting anything up to two weeks. This indicates that there is no national co-ordination of such courses and it is down to chance as to whether or not there is one in your area. If you are considering undertaking such a course you would perhaps be wise to discuss the course contents with the tutor to see if they match up with what you feel you need.

Should you be interviewed for a place in a return to nursing course the fact that you can indicate that you have been active in keeping up to date will be a positive point in your favour. This may increase your chances of not only a place on the course, but also a post with the employing authority. This keeping up to date may also go some way to avoid the feelings of low self-esteem and helplessness often expressed by nurses attempting to re-enter nursing following a break.

Registration

If you are an out of practice nurse who has intentions of returning to nursing at some stage, you would be well advised to maintain your registration as a nurse with the United Kingdom Central Council for Nursing Midwifery and Health Visiting. It is only through such registration that you have the legal right to practice as a registered nurse. Your registration lapses when there is non-payment of the three-year periodic fee and it involves time and money to have your name restored to the appropriate part of the register after its removal. There may be a temptation to let your registration lapse when on a break, but if you are engaged in updating on a regular basis then perhaps the relevance of maintaining your registration will be clearer.

Professional bodies

Like registration, the question of maintaining your membership of professional bodies and trade unions is well worth considering. This is particularly so if you belong to a body which organizes professional activities and courses and offers educational facilities. However, if you are paying fees just to ensure cover in the event of litigation and you do not make use of the organization's other facilities then the tendency to let the membership lapse will be strong. This could be short-sighted as you could maintain links with branch activities from time to time and thus have another valuable contact with working colleagues. That could help to lessen the alienation that seems to occur to nurses who are taking time out of their profession.

PERMANENT LEAVERS

Nurses leave nursing permanently for a number of different reasons and these include, leaving because the work was unsuitable or was physically too demanding, did not present enough of a challenge, or the financial rewards were too low and so on. However, a large number leave nursing permanently because they have reached the age of retirement and are required by their contract to terminate their employment.

Retirement

Retirement from work for many people may look an attractive proposition after many years of service. The thought of having more time to your self to do the things you have wanted to do and to be the master of your own life and dictate its pace is an exciting prospect. However, according to Rowe (1984) 'It has been suggested that approximately 75% of employed people say they look forward to approaching retirement. When it actually arrives only 30% say it was what they expected and that they are enjoying it.'

Thus merely dreaming about retirement and its possible benefits may not necessarily make them happen. Retirement has to be planned just as other life events have to be planned, for example getting married or starting a family or deciding on a career.

Pensions

This is probably the earliest and most important aspect of retirement planning as you have to be sure that you will have an adequate income during your retiral years, which can account for 30% of your life! For many nurses with unbroken careers the NHS superannuation scheme gives a useful retirement income in the shape of a lump sum and a monthly pension which, if fully matured by forty years of contributing reckonable service, could amount to half your normal monthly salary. This reckonable service can reach a maximum of 45 years if you work after the age of 60. Although this monthly pension is subject to income tax you do not pay national insurance or superannuation contributions. For nurses who have career breaks, the NHS superannuation scheme can also be of benefit as you can retain pension rights whilst out of the service. When contemplating a break in service, consult the personnel department to discuss the options open to you as a member of the superannuation scheme.

Many nurses have found themselves in less than favourable situations regards pension rights owing to the fact that they decided to withdraw their contributions when they left the service temporarily for the first time. They subsequently returned part-time and did not take the option of joining the scheme again, often to their regret. Protecting your super-annuation interests throughout the length of your career should be a priority for any nurse.

Nurses employed in the NHS usually retire between the ages of 55 and 60, although both men and women now have the opportunity to work to 65 if they so wish. For those in full-time employment, contributions to the NHS superannuation scheme would have been compulsory up until 6th April 1988. Due to the passing of the Social Security Act 1986, changes in the rules governing the NHS superannuation scheme occurred. A major change which came into effect on 6th April 1988, was that all Health Service employees who work more than half the standard full-time hours are entitled to choose whether or not they wish to remain members of the NHS superannuation scheme or opt to join another approved alternative scheme. The employees have to belong to some scheme, the changes merely allow choice. This means that you are free to negotiate a pension through an insurance company or to participate in the State Earnings-Related Pension Scheme, better known as SERPS. However, the basic state pension (old age pension) remains unaffected as the pensions mentioned above are intended to provide income over and above the state pension and not replace it.

Most pension experts would appear to advise those who have been with the NHS superannuation scheme for a number of years to remain with it as the final pension is index-linked (inflation proofed) and in the event of early retirement on the grounds of ill-health, years of service may be added to the final calculation of your pension. Such benefits as health cover and inflation proofing, in the private pension schemes, can be purchased at a price. Now that independent pension advice has become more available under the 1986 Social Security Act, it should be easier for nurses, interested in accumulating some extra capital for retirement, to do so with some confidence. Pension advisors have now to be independent of any insurance company or building society by law, and are required to give you the best possible unbiased advice regarding your purchasing of a pension. Such pension advice is usually free, but the advisor will be looking for your business. However, you should shop around for the best deal. A good pension advisor, should you decide to make a monthly investment to purchase a pension, should see you at least once a year and discuss how the investment is developing, it would be wise to check if this is part of the service. Nurses contributing to the NHS superannuation scheme do not get yearly consultations of this type as there is no investment in the same sense, but you can occasionally check to see just what benefits you have accrued. There are excellent booklets available on the superannuation scheme which may be obtained from the employing authority or from the appropriate superannuation office. The addresses of these offices appear at the end of this chapter.

Superannuation offices will also provide a detailed print-out about your benefits to date, all that is required to get this service is the completion of a simple form, usually available from the salaries department. This form is normally returned to the salaries department who will then send it to the superannuation office. Some employing authorities may have a salaries officer whose main job will be concerned with employee superannuation, thus expert advice may be found at this local source. Personnel departments can also give guidance on pension matters.

A pension paid from the NHS scheme is calculated by multiplying the member's final pay by the length of her service in years (days being expressed as a decimal fraction of a year) and dividing by eighty. The maximun service reckonable is normally 40 years by the age of 60 (55 for special cases, for example, mental health officers) and 45 years overall.

People not employed in superannuated jobs have to make their own arrangements for retirement income, over and above the state (old age) pension. They do this by taking out an insurance policy at an agreed premium and when it matures the money is used to buy a pension. This usually requires the expertise of a pension consultant to ensure the best return from the investment of the money.

Fit for retirement

If you have been used to working for a living for the best part of forty years then the question of replacement activity should perhaps be high on the agenda. Many people are heard to say that there will be 'plenty' to do during retiral, but seldom attempt to quantify it. Some think the small garden will keep them busy in retirement, only to find that it is possible to work in it for only seven or eight months in the year and that all that requires to be done can be accomplished in two days per week. Retirement and associated activities may need considerable thought and forward planning.

You may have to consider what is possible and much may depend on your state of health at the time of retiral and beyond. There is little doubt that, however you feel at the present, many will be subject to the normal processes of physical change as the retirement phase approaches. This does not imply helplessness, but it does require you to be realistic about the kinds of activities that can be engaged in, bearing in mind of course, that octagenarians have successfully run marathons!

This raises the issue of your own commitment to keeping fit and healthy during your working life, as this will increase your chances of reaching retirement in a reasonable physical state to enjoy it. Thus healthy living, along with pension arrangements, can be the start of long-term retiral planning.

Retirement should be seen as a change in one aspect of your life, namely employment, it need not involve wholesale withdrawal from associations, clubs or other groups. Most people are all too familiar with the individual who, on retirement, withdraws more or less from life. Returning from this state is usually always difficult. Some people who retire may actually take up alternative employment or become engaged in voluntary work until much later in their lives and hopefully, if this is employment, it is from free choice and not from necessity. Thus retirement should be regarded as a period of 'alternative engagement' rather than one of disengagement.

Pre-retirement courses

Employers are known, in some instances, to aid transition from work to retirement by offering employees the opportunity of attending a pre-retirement course. These courses can be run by the Health Service or by outside agencies. Work done by Anderson (1984) gave an example of a company who initiated the retiral preparation for its employees at the age of 50 and had follow-up courses at 55, 60 and 64. It is doubtful if the Health Service offers such an attractive pre-retiral package, but courses on the subject are becoming more available and are usually offered to employees in their last two years of employment. The fact that there are courses at all can be seen as an advance, as an investigation into the subject by Garrett (1983) revealed that less than 6% of the half million employees who retired in 1981 in the UK received any preparation for this change. Nurses who are beginning to plan their retirement should contact the personnel department and make enquires as to whether such courses are available, or are planned for the future.

Pre-retirement courses can be useful from a number of aspects. The input from the contributors involved in financial matters can prove most helpful, particularly when you consider that many who attend such courses will be shortly in receipt of fairly large lump sums of cash. The financial expert can explain some of the options that may be available should you wish to invest some of the pension cash. Indeed, from group discussion, a wide diversity of money related issues pertinent to retirement may be covered. This may give course members perspectives on retirement that may never have occurred to them.

The national health service fellowship

To newly retired nurses, the NHS Fellowship may be an organization that can offer much in the way of continuing interest and friendships. The Fellowship was formed in 1978 and now has in excess of 150 branches throughout the UK and over 16 000 members. It is an association of staff who have retired from the Health Service and includes their respective spouses.

The Fellowship exists to promote friendship and alleviate loneliness and worry amongst those who have retired from the Health Service. Branches decide on their own activities and how best the aims of the Fellowship can be met. Social events, speakers at monthly meetings, planned visits to retired and housebound colleagues and generally keeping members' interests to the fore, are the main activities. Information on where Fellowship branches are located can usually be obtained from personnel departments. The address of the central office is given at the end of the chapter.

When retirement becomes a reality this does not mean that your contribution to caring need necessarily end. For those wishing to do so, the question of voluntary work with hospitals, hospices or with the voluntary services may hold some attraction. In such situations you can feel you are continuing to make a useful contribution to society, that could be important to you. Whether you decide to keep an interest in nursing alive after retirement is obviously a personal choice, but continuing to meet with working colleagues from time to time at branch meetings of your professional body and maintaining your subscriptions to the journals, are ways of keeping in touch.

There is no doubt that thought and planning will aid the transition from working life to retirement and go a long way to ensuring that this is a satisfying and rewarding time of your life.

REFERENCES

Anderson, F. (1984) Retirement can damage your health. *Nursing Mirror*; **159**(3), 25–6.
Common Services Agency (1988) *Scottish Health Service Statistics*; Information and Statistics Divisional Publications, Edinburgh.
Donn, M. and Smits, M. (1988) Many happy returns. *Nursing Times*, **84**(47), 46–7.
Garrett, G. (1983) *Health Needs for the Elderly*, Macmillan, London.
Green, W. (1988) Making a comeback. *Nursing Times*, **84**(32), 50–1.
Mackay, I. (1988) Career women. *Nursing Times*, **84**(10), 42–4.
Melia, K. (1987) *Learning and Working: The Occupational Socialisation of Nurses*, Tavistock, London.
Rowe, M.J. (1984) Information for health now, with a happy retirement in view. *Health Libraries Review*, **1**(1), 11–6.
Waite, R. (1988) Most nurses will only go back part time. *Nursing Times*, **84**(14), 5.

FURTHER READING

Brown, P. (1988) Will you not come back again? *Nursing Times*, **84**(7), 44–5.
Chudley, P. (1988) Banking on retirement. *Nursing Standard*, **2**(22), 45.
Counsell, G. (1986) Getting to grips with pensions. *Physiotherapy*, **72**(8), 395.
Guntrip, G. (1985) Looking forward to retirement. *Nursing Mirror*, **161**(19), 32–3.
Heywood-Jones, I. (1986) *Back to Nursing with Confidence*, Heinemann, London.
Miller, H. (1978) *Countdown to Retirement*, Hutchinson Benham, London.
Morton-Cooper, A. (1988) Managing a successful return. *Nursing times*, **84**(7), 44–5.
Torrie, M. (1982) *Completing the Circle. New Ways of Life After Fifty*. Turnstone Press, Wellingborough.
Truman, C. (1987) Managing the career break, *Nursing Times*, **83**(3), 44–5.

USEFUL ADDRESSES

Department of Health and Social Security, Health Services Superannuation Division, Hesketh House Fleetwood, Lancashire FY7 8LG

Department of Health and Social Services, Health Services Superannuation Branch, 5a Fredrick Street, Belfast BT1 2LW

Scottish Office Superannuation Division, St Margaret's House, 151 London Road, Edinburgh EH8 7TG

National Health Service Retirement Fellowship, St Mary Abbots Hospital, Marloes Road, London W8 5LG

Index